ANTI-CANCER

A NEW WAY OF LIFE

Dr. Dustin M. Edwards

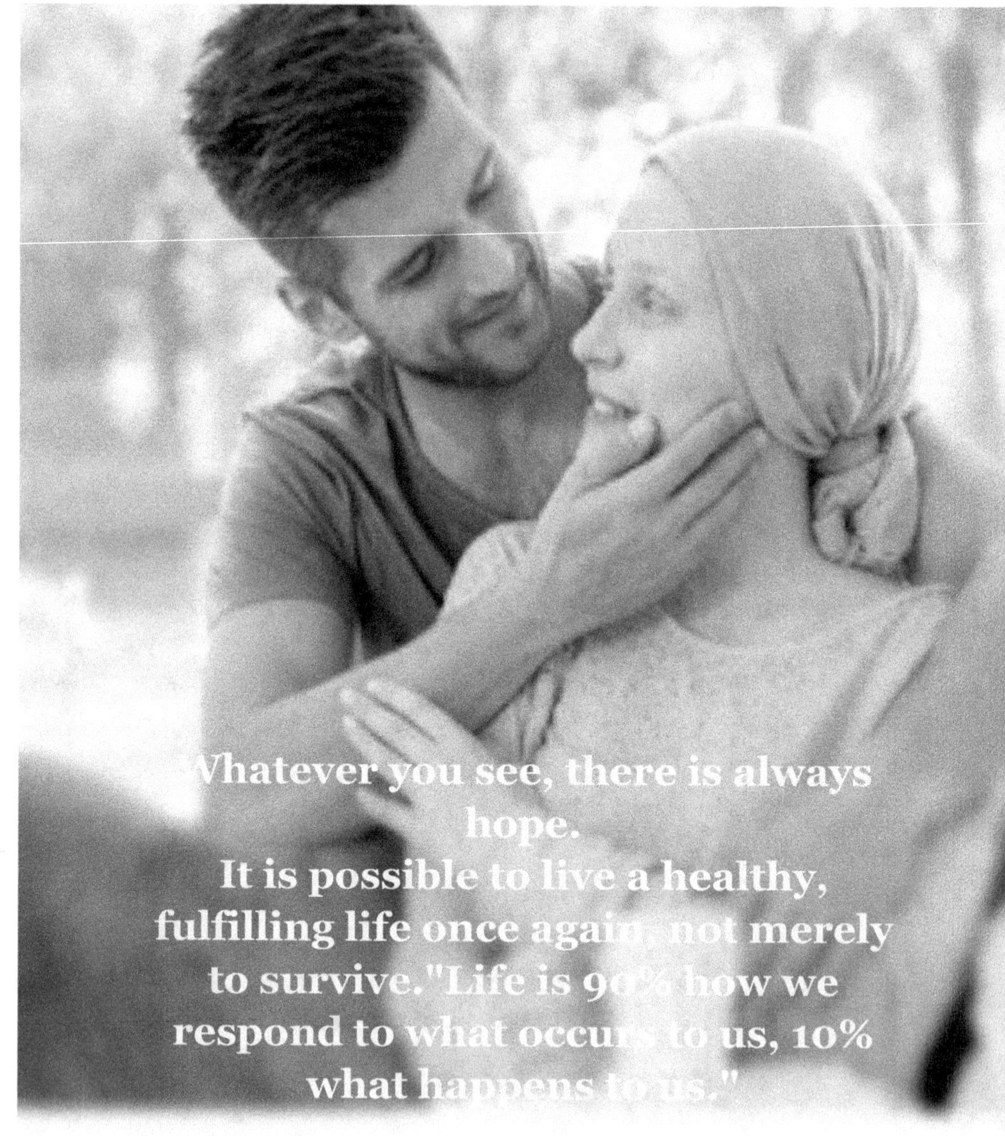

Whatever you see, there is always hope.
It is possible to live a healthy, fulfilling life once again, not merely to survive. "Life is 90% how we respond to what occurs to us, 10% what happens to us."

Table of content

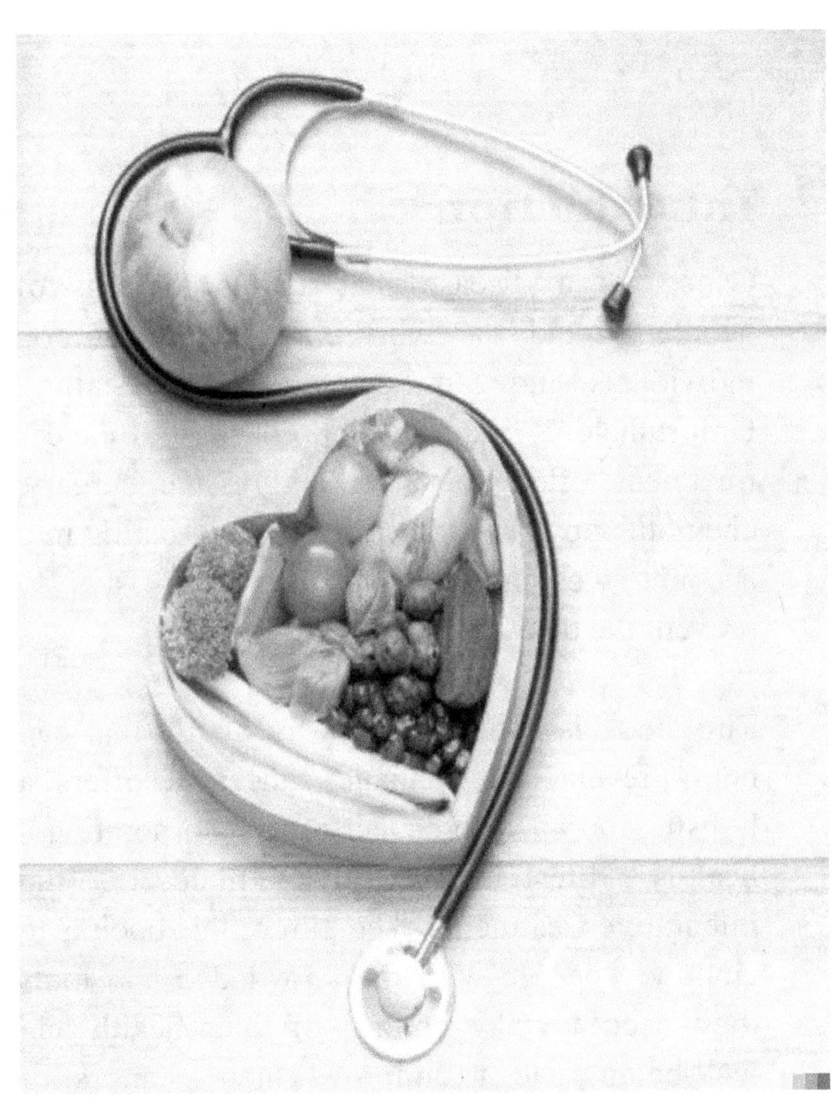

Introduction

Cancer is a disease that affects millions of people around the world, and its impact on individuals and families can be devastating. Unfortunately, traditional approaches to cancer treatment often focus on aggressive surgery, chemotherapy, and radiation, without taking into account the underlying causes and ways to prevent the disease.

This book is about a new way of life that can help prevent and manage cancer. It offers a holistic approach to cancer care, incorporating a healthy lifestyle, positive mindset, and integrative treatments. The aim of this book is to empower people with the knowledge and tools they need to take control of their health and well-being, and to improve their chances of surviving and thriving after a cancer diagnosis.

To illustrate the importance of this approach, we would like to share the story of Sarah, a cancer patient who suffered for a long time because of inappropriate treatment and a lack of understanding about cancer. Sarah was first diagnosed with breast cancer in her early 40s and underwent a mastectomy, followed by several rounds of chemotherapy and radiation. Despite her valiant efforts to beat the disease, the cancer returned and spread to other parts of her body.

Feeling helpless and hopeless, Sarah came across the first edition of this book and was inspired by its message of hope and empowerment. She made the decision to embrace the anti-cancer lifestyle, incorporating healthy eating, exercise, stress management, and alternative therapies into her treatment plan. To her great surprise and joy, Sarah found that her health improved dramatically, and she was able to beat the cancer into remission.

Sarah's story is a testament to the power of a positive attitude and a holistic approach to cancer care. By reading this book and embracing the anti-cancer lifestyle, you too can improve your chances of surviving and thriving after a cancer diagnosis. So let us begin this journey together and discover a new way of life that can help you overcome cancer and live a full, healthy life.

A. Purpose of the book

This book's goal is to provide readers a thorough and powerful manual for treating and avoiding cancer. Our mission is to empower people to take charge of their health and wellbeing, increase their chances of surviving and prospering after receiving a cancer diagnosis.

We consider cancer to be a complex illness that necessitates a multifaceted approach to treatment that includes both conventional and alternative therapies, as well as lifestyle modifications and a positive outlook. This book is intended to give readers the knowledge they need to comprehend the fundamental causes of cancer, how to prevent it, how to manage the condition, and how to enhance their quality of life in the event that they have already been diagnosed.

We cover a wide range of cancer-related topics in this book, including its origins, types, and stages of development as well as how it affects the body. Along with the significance of lifestyle modifications like stress reduction, healthy eating, exercise, and avoiding cancer-causing substances, we also talk about the importance of complementary and alternative therapies.

We also cover the mental and emotional effects of cancer, including how to deal with a cancer diagnosis, keep a positive outlook, and the value of support networks. We hope to equip readers with the information and resources they need to beat cancer and lead full, healthy lives by offering them a thorough and empowering guide to cancer care.

In a nutshell, the goal of this book is to educate readers on the causes of cancer as well as effective preventative and curative measures. People can take charge of their health, increase their chances of survival, and live a rich and fulfilling life even after receiving a cancer diagnosis by reading this book.

B. Overview of Cancer

Cancer is a group of diseases characterized by the uncontrolled growth and spread of abnormal cells in the body. It can affect virtually any part of the body, including the skin, bones, organs, and blood. Cancer is caused by mutations in the DNA of cells, which can occur spontaneously or as a result of exposure to environmental factors, such as tobacco smoke, radiation, or certain chemicals.

There are many different types of cancer, each of which affects different parts of the body and has different symptoms and prognosis. Some common types of cancer include breast cancer, lung cancer, prostate cancer, and colon cancer.

Cancer can be classified into different stages, depending on its severity and how far it has spread. In general, cancer is considered to be early stage if it is confined to its original location, and advanced stage if it has spread to other parts of the body.

The treatment of cancer typically involves a combination of conventional and alternative approaches, including surgery, chemotherapy, radiation, and immunotherapy, as well as complementary and alternative therapies, such as acupuncture, massage, and nutrition. The choice of treatment depends on the type and stage of the cancer, as well as the overall health and well-being of the patient.

The prognosis for cancer varies widely, depending on the type and stage of the disease, as well as the overall health and well-being of the patient. In general, early-stage cancers have a better prognosis than advanced-stage cancers, but with proper care and treatment, many people are able to overcome cancer and live full and satisfying lives.

In this book, we will explore the causes and types of cancer, as well as the various treatments and strategies for managing and preventing this disease. We will also discuss the importance of lifestyle changes, such as healthy eating, exercise, stress management, and avoiding cancer-causing substances, as well as the role of complementary and alternative therapies in cancer care. By understanding the nature of cancer and the various ways to manage and prevent it, individuals can take control of their health and improve their chances of survival and thriving after a cancer diagnosis.

C. The Need for a New Way of Life

Surgery, chemotherapy, and radiation have traditionally been the mainstays of the conventional cancer treatment strategy in order to remove or eradicate cancer cells. While these techniques sometimes work, they also have a number of negative side effects, such as discomfort, exhaustion, and a worse quality of life.

Additionally, the traditional method of treating cancer sometimes downplays the significance of dietary adjustments as well as complementary and alternative treatments, which may be quite helpful in the treatment and prevention of cancer. The conventional method of cancer therapy is just insufficient for many patients to recover from the illness and lead active, healthy lives.

When it comes to cancer, there is a growing understanding that we need a new way of life.

This new way of living entails adopting a holistic strategy for cancer treatment that includes both traditional and non-conventional therapies, as well as lifestyle adjustments and a positive outlook.

This new way of living is based on the idea that anybody can prevent and treat cancer by combining nutrition, exercise, stress management, avoiding drugs that cause cancer, and adopting complementary and alternative medicines. People may increase their chances of surviving and flourishing after receiving a cancer diagnosis by taking charge of their health and wellbeing.

This book is intended to help readers comprehend the need for a new way of living while dealing with cancer and to provide them with the knowledge they need to choose their own course of treatment. This book will provide you with the knowledge and resources you need to take charge of your health and lead a full, healthy life, whether you have been diagnosed with cancer or are just seeking for strategies to avoid this illness.

Chapter 1

Understanding Cancer

Understanding what cancer is and how it arises is crucial for the efficient management and prevention of the disease. A set of disorders known as cancer are defined by the body's aberrant cells growing and spreading out of control.

Genetic abnormalities, exposure to environmental variables like radiation and cigarette smoke, and lifestyle factors including an unhealthy diet, insufficient exercise, and excessive levels of stress are only a few of the causes of cancer.

There are several distinct forms of cancer, each of which impacts various bodily regions and has unique signs, symptoms, and prognoses. Breast cancer, lung cancer, prostate cancer, and colon cancer are a few typical cancers.

Healthcare professionals employ a range of examinations and imaging procedures, including biopsies, CT scans, and PET scans, to identify cancer. The kind and stage of the cancer, as well as the patient's general health and wellbeing, are taken into account when selecting a treatment strategy.

Cancer is often treated using a mix of traditional and unconventional methods, such as surgery, chemotherapy, radiation treatment, and immunotherapy, as well as complementary and unconventional therapies including acupuncture, massage, and diet.

The kind and stage of the cancer, as well as the patient's general health and wellbeing, all have a significant impact on the prognosis. Although early-stage cancers often have a better prognosis than advanced-stage cancers, many patients may beat the disease and lead fulfilling lives with the right care and therapy.

We will go more deeply into the nature of cancer in this chapter of the book, including its causes, forms, and symptoms. Additionally, we'll talk about the numerous cancer diagnostic procedures and cancer management and prevention strategies. People may take charge of their health, increase their chances of surviving and flourishing after a cancer diagnosis, and take charge of their health by knowing cancer and the many management and prevention techniques.

A. Causes of Cancer

Cancer is a complex and multifaceted disease that can be caused by a variety of factors. Some of the most common causes of cancer include:

1. Genetics

A person with familial adenomatous polyposis has many colon polyps.

Despite the fact that there are more than 50 hereditary cancers that can be distinguished, only 0.3% of people have a genetic mutation that increases the risk of developing cancer, and these instances account for just 3–10% of all cancer cases.

Most malignancies are not inherited ("sporadic cancers").

An inherited genetic flaw is the main cause of hereditary malignancies. An inherited genetic mutation in one or more genes predisposes the afflicted persons to the development of malignancies and may also cause the early start of these diseases. This condition is known as cancer syndrome or familial cancer syndrome. Cancer risk varies, even though cancer syndromes show an elevated risk. Cancer is an uncommon side effect of several of these disorders and is not their main characteristic.

Mutations in tumor suppressor genes, which control cell development, are the primary cause of many cancer syndrome cases. The activity of oncogenes, DNA repair genes, and genes involved in blood vessel development are all affected by other frequent mutations. Breast cancer and ovarian cancer risk is increased by certain hereditary mutations in the BRCA1 and BRCA2 genes by more than 75%. Familial adenomatous polyposis and hereditary non-polyposis colon cancer are two examples of inherited genetic abnormalities that may cause colorectal cancer, though they account for fewer than 5% of cases. Genetic testing is often used to find altered genes or chromosomes that are handed down through the generations.

Depending on the kind of cell in which they manifest, gene mutations are categorized as either germline or somatic (germline cells include the egg and the sperm and somatic cells are those forming the body). The risk of cancer is raised by the germline mutations, which are passed down through generations.

2. Chemical and physical irritants

Smoking and cancer, carcinogens, and safety of e-cigarettes

Certain compounds, known as carcinogens, have been associated with certain cancer forms. Inhaled asbestos, certain dioxins, and cigarette smoke are typical examples of non-radioactive carcinogens. Carcinogenicity may occur in both natural and synthetic compounds, despite the prevalent public perception that it only occurs in synthetic chemicals.

Occupation is thought to be responsible for 20,000 cancer deaths and 40,000 new instances of cancer each year in the United States. At least 200,000 individuals worldwide pass away from cancer connected to their line of employment each year. Millions of employees are at danger of contracting leukemia from exposure to benzene at work or lung cancer and mesothelioma from cigarette smoke and asbestos fibers, respectively.

An estimated 2 to 20% of all instances of cancer are thought to be connected to a person's line of work. The developed world is where occupational risk factors account for the majority of cancer fatalities. At least for lung, colorectal, breast, and prostate cancers, job stress does not seem to be a substantial risk factor. Due to exposure to the chemical 2,4-D, taking part in Operation Ranchhand in Vietnam during the Vietnam War, living on a golf course, or working on a farm would all raise your chance of developing non-Hodgkins lymphoma. Agent Orange is the name given to the mixture of 2,4-D and 2,4-T, two chemical pesticides or herbicides, when blended in a 50:50 ratio.

i. Smoke

Smoking and the risk of developing lung cancer are closely associated.

80% of lung cancers are brought on by tobacco use, which is linked to many other types of cancer.

The association between smoking and cancers of the lung, larynx, head, neck, stomach, bladder, kidney, esophagus, and pancreas has been shown by decades of study.

The risk of myeloid leukemia, squamous cell sinonasal cancer, liver cancer, colorectal cancer, malignancies of the gallbladder, adrenal gland, small intestine, and several children cancers may be somewhat elevated, according to some research.

The toxicants in cigarette smoke that are most often linked to the development of respiratory tract cancer have been identified as seven.
Two of these, acrylonitrile and acrolein, seem to have oxidative stress and oxidative DNA damage as part of their mechanisms of action.

Acetaldehyde, cadmium, ethylene oxide, formaldehyde, and isoprene are the other five toxicants. They exert their effects by a variety of methods, including direct DNA contact. More than fifty recognized carcinogens, including nitrosamines and polycyclic aromatic hydrocarbons, are found in tobacco smoke. Around one in five cancer deaths globally and one in three in the industrialized world are caused by tobacco. In the United States, lung cancer death rates have followed a similar trend to that of smoking, with smoking rates rising followed by sharp rises in lung cancer death rates, and more recently, smoking rates falling since the 1950s followed by falls in male lung cancer death rates since 1990. Nevertheless, the global smoking rate is still increasing, contributing to what some groups have dubbed the tobacco pandemic.

Electronic cigarettes, often known as e-cigarettes, are portable electronic gadgets that mimic the sensation of smoking tobacco. Daily, long-term use of high voltage electronic cigarettes may produce more formaldehyde-forming compounds than smoking, which was shown to have a 5 to 15-fold higher lifetime cancer risk than smoking. However, it is still unclear how safe they are generally and what long-term health impacts they will have.

ii. Materials

A cytological slide with an asbestos body

Some toxins mainly affect cells physically, as opposed to chemically, to induce cancer.

Long-term exposure to asbestos, which are naturally occurring mineral fibers, is a notable illustration of this. Mesothelioma is a cancer of the serous membrane, most often the serous membrane around the lungs.

Wollastonite, attapulgite, glass wool, and rock wool are among the compounds in this group that are thought to have effects that are comparable to those of asbestos.

Powdered metallic cobalt, nickel, and crystalline silica are non-fibrous particle cancer-causing substances (quartz, cristobalite, and tridymite).

Physical carcinogens often need to enter the body (for example, by microscopic fragments being inhaled) and be exposed for years before cancer may form.

3. Personal habits Alcohol and cancer, obesity and cancer, and diet

Several distinct lifestyle choices raise the chance of developing cancer. About 30–35% of cancer mortality are linked with obesity and nutrition. The majority of dietary guidelines for the prevention of cancer place a focus on fruits, vegetables, whole grains, and seafood while advising against processed meat, red meat, animal fats, and refined carbs. These dietary modifications are supported by some but not conclusive data.

i. Liquor

Alcohol abuse may cause liver cirrhosis (seen above) and hepatocellular carcinoma, a kind of liver cancer, by causing chronic liver damage.

One example of a chemical carcinogen is alcohol. Alcohol has been categorized by the World Health Organization as a Group 1 carcinogen. Alcohol is blamed for 10% of male malignancies and 3% of female cancers in Western Europe.

Alcohol is a factor in 3.6% of all cancer cases and 3.5% of cancer-related deaths worldwide. The chance of acquiring malignancies of the mouth, esophagus, pharynx, larynx, stomach, liver, ovaries, and colon has been proven to be increased by alcohol usage in particular. Increased exposure to the carcinogen and breakdown product of ethanol, acetaldehyde, plays a major role in the development of cancer. DNA interstrand crosslinks, a kind of DNA damage, are brought on by acetaldehyde. A flawed replication-coupled DNA repair mechanism may correct them.

Increased mutation frequency and a modified mutational spectrum are the effects of this repair process. Other explanations have been put up, such as nutritional inadequacies brought on by alcohol, changes to DNA methylation, and the development of oxidative stress in tissues.

ii. Diet

Certain foods have been connected to certain malignancies. According to studies, those who consume red or processed meat are more likely to get pancreatic, prostate, and breast cancer. The presence of carcinogens in food cooked at high temperatures may help to partly explain this. High fat intake, alcohol consumption, consumption of red and processed meats, obesity, and inactivity are a few risk factors for colorectal cancer. Gastric cancer is associated with a high-salt diet. A common dietary contaminant called aflatoxin B1 has been linked to liver cancer. Oral cancer has been linked to eating betel nuts.

Different cancer incidence rates in various nations may be partially explained by the connection between food and the development of certain tumors. For instance, colon cancer is more prevalent in the United States owing to the increasing consumption of processed and red meat, but stomach cancer is more frequent in Japan due to the frequency of high-salt diets. Within one to two generations, immigrant populations often adopt the country's cancer risk profile, indicating a strong connection between food and cancer.

45% to 56% of mice got colon cancer over the course of the next 10 months when deoxycholate was given to their food to the same extent as deoxycholate was found in the feces of humans on a high fat diet. In contrast, none of the mice on a diet without deoxycholate acquired cancer.

Circulating deoxycholate as well as other particular bile acids and the risk of colorectal cancer in women are strongly correlated, according to a new prospective human research looking at the connection between microbial metabolites and cancer.

iii. Overweight

In the United States, being overweight is linked to the emergence of several cancer types and contributes to 14–20% of all cancer-related fatalities.

In the US, obesity is a factor in almost 85,000 new cancer diagnoses each year.

Cancer incidence and death have decreased in those who had bariatric surgery for weight reduction.

Obesity is linked to esophageal, endometrial, renal, and post-menopausal breast cancers as well as colon and post-menopausal breast cancer.

Additionally, liver cancer has been linked to obesity.

According to current theories, aberrant amounts of sex hormones and metabolic proteins, notably insulin-like growth factors, contribute to the development of cancer in obese people (estrogens, androgens and progestogens).

Additionally, adipose tissue fosters an inflammatory environment that may aid in the growth of malignancies.

Dysregulation of adipose tissue may cause oxidative stress, which damages DNA and increases the risk of cancer.

Physical inactivity is thought to increase the risk of cancer not just through affecting body weight but also by having a detrimental impact on the immunological and endocrine systems.

Instead of being caused by eating too few healthful foods, overnutrition accounts for more than half of the effects of diet.

4. Hormones

breast invasive ductal carcinoma as seen under the microscope. The yellow, healthy fatty tissue surrounds the pale, crab-shaped lump that is the tumor.

Some hormones encourage cell proliferation, which contributes to the development of cancer.

Insulin-like growth factors and their binding proteins are essential for the proliferation, differentiation, and death of cancer cells, indicating a potential role in the development of cancer.

In sex-related malignancies such those of the breast, endometrial, prostate, ovary, and testis, as well as thyroid cancer and bone cancer, hormones play a significant role.

For instance, daughters of breast cancer survivors had much greater levels of estrogen and progesterone than daughters of breast cancer survivors. Even in the absence of a breast-cancer gene, these women may have an increased chance of developing breast cancer due to these elevated hormone levels. Similar to this, men of African heritage have much greater testosterone levels than men of European ancestry, and as a result, their rates of prostate cancer are also significantly higher. Asian men had the lowest rates of prostate cancer due to their androstanediol glucuronide levels, which activate testosterone.

Obese persons have greater levels of several hormones linked to cancer and a higher incidence of those tumors, which are additional variables that are important.

Hormone replacement treatment users are more likely to develop malignancies linked to those hormones.

Contrarily, those who exercise more than the usual amount have lower levels of these hormones and a decreased chance of developing cancer.

Growth hormones may encourage osteosarcoma.

Some medical procedures and preventative measures make advantage of this situation by artificially lowering hormone levels, which deters the development of malignancies that are hormone-sensitive. Changes in the amounts or activity of certain hormones may cause some malignancies to stop growing or even experience cell death since steroid hormones are potent regulators of gene expression in some cancer cells. The use of the selective estrogen-receptor modulator tamoxifen for the treatment of breast cancer is perhaps the most well-known instance of hormonal therapy in oncology. Aromatase inhibitors, a different family of hormonal drugs, are increasingly playing a larger part in the management of breast cancer.

5. Inflammation and infection cancerous infections: causes

Cancerous infections have a role in around 18% of cancer cases worldwide. This percentage fluctuates around the globe, reaching a high of 25% in Africa and falling to under 10% in the industrialized world. The typical infectious agents that cause cancer are viruses, although parasites and bacteria also play a role. Genomic instability or DNA damage are typical causes of cancer risk-raising infectious organisms.

i: viruses

The most prevalent virus that affects the reproductive system is HPV. Cervical cancer in women may occur as a result of infection.

A significant risk factor for liver and cervical cancer is viral infection. An oncovirus is a kind of virus that may cause cancer. These include the hepatitis B and hepatitis C viruses (hepatocellular carcinoma), human papillomavirus (cervical carcinoma), Epstein-Barr virus (B-cell lymphoproliferative disease and nasopharyngeal carcinoma), Kaposi's sarcoma herpesvirus (Kaposi's sarcoma and primary effusion lymphomas), and human T-cell leukemia virus-1 (T-cell leukemias).

The three most prevalent oncoviruses in Western industrialized nations are the human papillomavirus (HPV), hepatitis B virus (HBV), and hepatitis C virus (HCV). The majority of cervical cancers, as well as certain cancers of the vagina, vulva, penis, anus, rectum, throat, tongue, and tonsils, are all brought on by HPV in the United States. The HPV E6 and E7 oncoproteins among high-risk HPV viruses inactivate tumor suppressor genes when they infect cells.

Additionally, the oncoproteins independently cause genomic instability in healthy human cells, which raises the chance of developing cancer. More than 200 times as many people with chronic hepatitis B virus infection will develop liver cancer as those who are not infected. The development of liver cancer is independently linked to liver cirrhosis, whether brought on by chronic viral hepatitis infection or heavy alcohol use, although the risk is greatest when both conditions are present.

ii. Parasites and bacteria

Schistosoma haematobium eggs in the bladder lining: histopathology.

As observed in gastric carcinoma caused by Helicobacter pylori, other bacterial infections may potentially raise the chance of developing cancer. Chronic inflammation or the direct action of certain of the bacteria's virulence proteins may play a role in how H. pylori promotes cancer. Schistosoma haematobium (squamous cell carcinoma of the bladder) and the liver flukes Opisthorchis viverrini and Clonorchis sinensis are parasitic illnesses that are closely linked to cancer (cholangiocarcinoma). The worm's eggs seem to be the mechanism that causes inflammation, which in turn causes cancer. Additionally, certain parasite infections may increase the amount of cancer-causing substances in the body, which can result in the growth of malignancies. Lung cancer development has also been connected to TB infection, which is brought on by the mycobacterium M. tuberculosis.

iii. An infection

There is evidence that inflammation contributes significantly to the initiation and spread of cancer. Chronic inflammation has the potential to cause DNA deterioration over time as well as the buildup of random genetic mutations in cancer cells. By affecting the tumor microenvironment, inflammation may aid in the growth, survival, angiogenesis, and migration of cancer cells. A higher risk of colorectal cancer exists in those with inflammatory bowel illness.

6. Radiation Cancer brought on by radiation

Radiation exposure, including both ionizing and non-ionizing radiation, is linked to up to 10% of invasive malignancies.

In contrast to physical or chemical causes of cancer, ionizing radiation randomly affects cellular molecules. If a chromosome is struck, it may break, produce an aberrant number of chromosomes, inactivate one or more genes in that portion of the chromosome, erase portions of the DNA sequence, result in chromosomal translocations, or result in other chromosome abnormalities. Smaller damage may leave a stable, partially functioning cell that may be capable of replicating and growing into cancer, particularly if tumor suppressor genes were damaged by the radiation.

Major damage often results in the cell dying. Ionizing radiation seems to cause cancer in three distinct stages: morphological alterations to the cell, cellular immortality (loss of normal, life-limiting cell regulatory systems), and adaptations that promote tumor growth. Even if the radiation particle doesn't directly hit the

40

DNA, it still causes reactions in the cells that subtly raise the risk of mutations.

Non-ionizing radiation, first
Squamous cell cancer on the nose's sun-exposed skin.

Electromagnetic radiation is not always cancer-causing. It is believed that low-energy electromagnetic waves, such as radio waves, microwaves, infrared radiation, and visible light, are not because they lack the energy to dissolve chemical bonds. The International Agency for Research on Cancer of the World Health Organization has classified non-ionizing radio frequency radiation from electric power transmission, mobile phones, and other comparable sources as a potential carcinogen. Studies, however, have not consistently linked cancer risk to mobile phone radiation.

Higher energy radiation, such as gamma, x, and ultraviolet radiation (found in sunlight), is often cancer-causing if ingested in high enough levels.

Melanoma and other skin cancers may develop from long-term sun exposure to UV light. Non-melanoma skin cancers are the majority of non-invasive malignancies that are brought on by non-ionizing UV radiation. The majority of non-melanoma skin cancers, which are the most prevalent types of cancer in the world, are shown to be caused by ultraviolet radiation, particularly the non-ionizing medium wave UVB.

Ionizing radiation, second

Meningioma displacement of the underlying brain in cross section.

Medical imaging and radon gas are two sources of ionizing radiation. The mutagen effect of ionizing radiation is not very significant. Radiation-induced malignancies are increasingly being caused by the use of ionizing radiation in medicine. Ionizing radiation may be used to treat various malignancies, but in certain situations, it may also result in the development of a different kind of cancer. Although radiation-induced solid tumors normally take 10-15 years to develop clinically and may take up to 40 years to exhibit, and radiation-induced leukemias typically take 2–10 years to display, radiation can cause cancer in various body areas, in all species, and at any age. A rare side effect of cranial irradiation is meningiomas caused by radiation.

Some individuals are more likely than usual to get cancer from radiation exposure, such as those with retinoblastoma or nevoid basal cell carcinoma syndrome. Radiation exposure before birth has ten times the impact and increases the risk of radiation-induced leukemia in children and adolescents compared to adults.

Some types of medical imaging also employ ionizing radiation. Medical imaging exposes the population to radiation doses that are nearly as high as background radiation in developed nations. Using nuclear medical procedures, radioactive drugs are injected straight into the circulation.

As a kind of illness treatment, radiotherapy purposefully administers high doses of radiation to malignancies and surrounding tissues. According to estimates, 0.4% of cancer cases in the US in 2007 were brought on by earlier CT scans, and this number might rise to 1.5–2% if CT use rates grow over the same timeframe.

As with passive smoking, radon gas exposure in homes increases the chance of developing cancer.

It is widely accepted that low-dose exposures, such as living close to a nuclear power station, have little or very little impact on the development of cancer.

When paired with other cancer-causing factors, such as exposure to radon gas and cigarette use, radiation is a more powerful cause of cancer.

7. Unusual causes

It is very uncommon for donor-derived cancers to form after organ donations. Malignant melanoma that was undiagnosed at the time of organ harvest seems to be the primary contributor to malignancies linked with organ transplants. Virus-infected donor cells have also been linked to cases of Kaposi's sarcoma developing following transplantation.

i: trauma

Cancer caused by physical trauma is rather uncommon. For instance, it has never been established that shattering bones causes bone cancer. Similar to how physical trauma is not recognized as a cause of brain, breast, or cervical cancer. Regular, sustained application of hot items to the body is one recognized cause. Repeated burns to the same area of the body, such those caused by charcoal hand warmers like the kanger and kairo, have the potential to cause skin cancer, particularly if other carcinogenic substances are also present.

Drinking scalding hot tea often might cause esophageal cancer.

In general, it is thought that rather than being immediately brought on by the trauma, cancer develops or a pre-existing cancer is promoted throughout the healing process. But if the same tissues are injured repeatedly, this would encourage excessive cell growth, which would raise the likelihood of a malignant mutation.

ii. Transmission from mother to fetus

Acute leukemia, lymphoma, melanoma, and carcinoma have been observed to be transmitted transplacentally from the mother to the fetus in the United States, where 3,500 pregnant women are diagnosed with a malignancy each year. Cancer is often not a transmissible illness, with the exception of the very uncommon transmissions that happen during pregnancy and only a very small number of organ donors. This is mostly due to tissue transplant rejection brought on by MHC incompatibility. Because

MHC antigens vary from person to person, the immune system employs them in humans and other vertebrates to distinguish between "self" and "non-self" cells. The immune system responds against the correct cell when non-self antigens are met. By removing inserted cells, such responses may prevent tumor cell engraftment.

B. Symptoms of cancer

There are many different types of symptoms base on the type of cancer. Some individuals have unusual pimples, fevers that are not explained, nocturnal sweats, or unintended weight loss.

BREAST CANCER SYMPTOMS

Lumps or thickening in the breast or underarm, change in size or shape of the breast, dimpling or puckering of the skin on the breast, redness or scaliness of the nipple or breast skin, fluid discharge from the nipple, pain or tenderness in the Breast cancer warning indicators include:breast.Lumps or thickening in the breast or underarm, change in size or shape of the breast, dimpling or puckering of the skin on the breast, redness or scaliness of the nipple or breast skin, fluid discharge from the nipple, pain or tenderness in the breast.

COMMON SIGNS

1. A new breast or underarm lump (armpit).
2. An area of the breast that has thickened or enlarged.
3. Dimpling or irritation of the breast skin.
4. Nipple or breast region redness or dry skin.
5. Nipple pulling in or soreness in the nipple region.
6. Nipple discharge, including blood, that is not breast milk.
7. Any modification to the breast's size or form.
8. Aches in any breast location.

Causes: Family history of breast cancer, personal history of breast cancer, exposure to radiation, increasing age, early onset of menstrual periods, late menopause, having no children or having children after age 30, obesity, alcohol consumption, hormonal therapy for menopause.

PROSTATE CANCER SYMPTOMS

In its early stages, prostate cancer may not show any symptoms at all.

More advanced prostate cancer may exhibit symptoms and indications like:

1. Urinary issues
2. Less force in the urine stream
3. Urine with blood in it
4. Semen with blood in it
5. Bone aches
6. Weight loss without effort
7. Irregular erections

Causes: Age, family history of prostate cancer, African-American race, obesity, a high-fat diet, exposure to cadmium.

BASAL CELL CANCERS SYMPTOMS

Almost all basal cell carcinomas (BCCs) may be effectively removed without problems with early identification and treatment. One or more of the symptoms is:

1. An unhealed open sore that may bleed, leak, or crust. It's possible for the discomfort to last for weeks or for it to seem to heal before returning.

2. An inflamed or reddish spot on the face, chest, shoulder, arm, or leg that may crust, itch, pain, or not be at all uncomfortable.

3. A pearly, clear, pink, red, or white shining protrusion or nodule. The bump might resemble a typical mole if it is tan, black, or brown, particularly among persons of race.

4. A little pink growth that is crusted in the center and has a raised, rolling edge. Over time, it may produce a few surface blood vessels.

5. An region that resembles a scar and is waxy, yellow, or flat white in appearance. The skin looks tight and glossy, with sometimes

ill-defined boundaries. This cautionary indication can point to an intrusive BCC.

C. Types of Cancer

There are many different types of cancer, each of which affects different parts of the body and has different symptoms and prognoses. Some of the most common types of cancer include:

1. Carcinomas: Carcinomas are the most common type of cancer and are characterized by the uncontrolled growth of cells in the epithelial tissue, which makes up the skin and the lining of organs and glands. Examples of carcinomas include breast cancer, lung cancer, and prostate cancer.

2. Sarcomas: Sarcomas are a type of cancer that affects the connective tissue, such as bones, muscles, and cartilage. Examples of sarcomas include osteosarcoma and chondrosarcoma.

3. Leukemias: Leukemias are a type of cancer that affects the blood-forming cells, such as white blood cells and red blood cells. Examples of leukemias include acute lymphoblastic leukemia (ALL) and acute myeloid leukemia (AML).

4. Lymphomas: Lymphomas are a type of cancer that affects the lymphatic system, including the lymph nodes and other organs. Examples of lymphomas include Hodgkin's lymphoma and non-Hodgkin's lymphoma.

5. Central Nervous System Cancers: Central nervous system cancers are a type of cancer that affects the brain and spinal cord. Examples of central nervous system cancers include glioblastoma and medulloblastoma

6. Melanoma: Melanoma is a type of skin cancer that is characterized by the uncontrolled growth of pigment-producing cells in the skin. Examples of melanoma include malignant melanoma and nodular melanoma.

7. Gastrointestinal Cancers: Gastrointestinal cancers are a type of cancer that affects the digestive system, including the esophagus, stomach, small intestine, colon, and rectum. Examples of gastrointestinal cancers include colon cancer, rectal cancer, and gastric cancer.

8. Gynecologic Cancers: Gynecologic cancers are a type of cancer that affects the female reproductive system, including the uterus, ovaries, and cervix. Examples of gynecologic cancers include ovarian cancer, uterine cancer, and cervical cancer.

9. Genitourinary Cancers: Genitourinary cancers are a type of cancer that affects the urinary and reproductive systems, including the bladder, kidney, and testicles. Examples of genitourinary cancers include bladder cancer, kidney cancer, and testicular cancer.

10. Thyroid Cancer: Thyroid cancer is a type of cancer that affects the thyroid gland, a small gland located at the base of the neck that produces hormones that regulate the body's metabolism. Examples of thyroid cancer include papillary thyroid cancer and follicular thyroid cancer.

11. Blood Cancers: Blood cancers are a type of cancer that affects the blood cells, including the white blood cells, red blood cells, and platelets. Examples of blood cancers include acute lymphoblastic leukemia (ALL), acute myeloid leukemia (AML), and multiple myeloma.

The specific treatment plan for each type of cancer will depend on the stage and location of the cancer, as well as the patient's overall health and medical history. Some types of cancer may be treated with surgery, radiation therapy, chemotherapy, or a combination of these treatments. Other types of cancer may be treated with more targeted therapies, such as immunotherapy or hormone therapy.

It is important for individuals to be aware of the different types of cancer and to seek medical attention if they notice any symptoms or changes in their health. Early detection is key in increasing the chances of a successful treatment outcome, and can make a significant difference in the prognosis and survival rate for individuals with cancer.

In this section of the book, we will take a closer look at each of the different types of cancer and explore the various causes, symptoms, and treatments for each type. We will also delve into the latest research and advances in cancer treatment, and explore how these treatments are helping individuals and families to fight cancer and reclaim their lives.

D. Stages of Cancer Development

The stages of cancer development describe how far a cancer has progressed and help determine the best course of treatment. The most commonly used cancer staging system is the TNM system, which stands for Tumor, Node, Metastasis. The TNM system considers the size of the primary tumor, the presence of cancer cells in nearby lymph nodes, and whether the cancer has spread to distant parts of the body.

Stage 0: This is the earliest stage of cancer, where abnormal cells are present but have not spread beyond the original location.

Stage I: In this stage, the cancer is still small and contained within the primary site. It may have grown into nearby tissues but has not spread to the lymph nodes.

Stage II: The cancer is larger and may have spread to nearby lymph nodes, but it has not spread to other parts of the body.

Stage III: The cancer has spread to nearby lymph nodes and may have also spread to other parts of the body, but it is still contained within a limited area.

Stage IV: This is the most advanced stage of cancer, where the cancer has spread to distant parts of the body and may have formed secondary tumors in other organs.

It is important to note that the staging of cancer can change as a person undergoes treatment or the cancer progresses. The staging is a crucial part of the diagnostic process, as it helps determine the best course of treatment and provides a baseline for monitoring the effectiveness of treatment over time. The stage of cancer also helps predict the likelihood of recovery and survival.

The stages of cancer development can be determined through a variety of diagnostic tests, including:

Physical examination: Your doctor will conduct a thorough physical examination to check for any signs or symptoms of cancer.

Imaging tests: These may include X-rays, CT scans, MRI scans, PET scans, and other imaging tests that create pictures of the inside of your body. These tests can help determine the size and location of a tumor and whether it has spread to other parts of the body.

Biopsy: A biopsy is a procedure in which a small sample of tissue is removed from the body and examined under a microscope. This is the only way to definitively diagnose cancer.

Blood tests: Blood tests can be used to check for elevated levels of certain markers that are associated with cancer, such as the presence of cancer cells or specific proteins produced by cancer cells.

Staging tests: Once a cancer diagnosis has been confirmed, your doctor may conduct additional tests to determine the stage of your cancer. This may include further imaging tests, such as a bone scan or a liver function test, or the removal of additional tissue samples for examination.

Your doctor will use the results of these tests to determine the stage of your cancer and develop an appropriate treatment plan. It is important to work closely with your doctor to understand your diagnosis and the available treatment options. Early detection and prompt treatment can greatly improve the chances of a positive outcome.

E. The Impact of Cancer on the Body

Cancer can have a significant impact on the body, both physically and emotionally. The effects of cancer and its treatment can vary depending on the type of cancer, its stage, and the person's overall health. *Some of the ways cancer can impact the body include:*

Physical symptoms: Depending on the location and stage of the cancer, a person may experience pain, fatigue, weight loss, changes in appetite, and other physical symptoms.

Treatment side effects: Cancer treatment, including surgery, chemotherapy, and radiation therapy, can cause a wide range of side effects, including nausea, vomiting, hair loss, and changes in skin appearance.

Cognitive effects: Cancer and its treatment can also affect cognitive function, leading to problems with memory, attention, and concentration.

Physical limitations: Depending on the type and stage of cancer, a person may experience physical limitations that affect their ability to perform daily activities and their overall quality of life.

Cancer may alter your body's regular chemical balance and raise your risk of life-threatening problems. Chemical imbalances may show symptoms such as increased thirst, frequent urination, constipation, and disorientation. issues with the nerve system and brain.

Social and Emotional Effects of cancer

Nearly all cancer patients will have psychological and emotional problems, which may manifest years after therapy. You do not have to go through this alone, which is wonderful news. You have access to community services, social media, therapy, and support groups to assist you deal with these problems. Realizing you have a problem and having the confidence to ask for assistance are the first steps in dealing with psychosocial changes.

The following are some of the most typical psychological problems that cancer patients may experience:

1. Fear of recurrence: Many cancer survivors are concerned that their disease may eventually return. These emotions are often brought on by significant moments in their cancer experience. Understanding your own body might make it easier to differentiate between typical bodily changes and more worrisome symptoms that should be reported to your doctor.

Loss naturally leads to grief. Loss might affect your physical independence, fertility, sex desire, and health. You may work through these challenges with the aid of support groups and therapy.

Depression: It's thought that 70% of cancer survivors will go through periods of depression. Recognize the signs of depression and get help as soon as you can.

Body image: Cancer patients who have had amputations, deformity, or a significant alteration in their physical function may have low self-esteem. Your desire for closeness and social contact may be impacted by a bad body image. Positive emotions may be reduced by open, honest dialogue with loved ones.

Spirituality: After a cancer diagnosis, many survivors discover that life has new meaning and decide to recommit to organized religion or spiritual pursuits. According to research, having a strong social support system, learning new coping mechanisms, feeling less depressed, and having improved physical health all contribute to higher quality of life.

Some individuals feel guilty for surviving cancer whereas others don't. Seek assistance from a psychologist, a clergyperson, or a support group if you have a persistent sensation of guilt.

Relationships: Following a cancer diagnosis, you could notice that friends, colleagues, and family members approach you differently. They could shun you or refuse to ask about your disease. Seeking out new connections with cancer survivors who have experienced similar things to you might be beneficial.

Workplace: Cancer survivors often feel that they are no longer able to connect to their coworkers who have not been affected by the disease. Because you don't want to be treated unfairly, you may be hesitant to discuss your cancer treatment with colleagues or your job. Check to see whether your company offers a cancer survivorship support group or other services.

It is important to understand the potential impact of cancer on the body and to work with a healthcare team to manage symptoms and side effects. There are many support services and resources available to help people with cancer, including therapy, support groups, and physical rehabilitation. By working together, people with cancer and their healthcare providers can develop a plan to manage the physical and emotional effects of cancer and improve overall well-being.

Chapter 2

Prevention is Key

The old saying "prevention is key" holds especially true when it comes to cancer. There are many things that individuals can do to reduce their risk of developing cancer and to improve their chances of detecting it early, when it is most treatable. Here are a few key ways to prevent cancer:

Live a Healthy Lifestyle: Eating a healthy, balanced diet, getting regular physical activity, maintaining a healthy weight, avoiding tobacco, and limiting alcohol consumption are all important ways to reduce your risk of developing cancer.

Get Screened Regularly: Screening tests can detect cancer early, when it is most treatable. Examples of screening tests for different types of cancer include mammograms for breast cancer, colonoscopies for colorectal cancer, and PSA tests for prostate cancer. Talk to your doctor about which screening tests are right for you and how often you should get them.

Avoid Exposure to Harmful Substances: Exposure to certain chemicals and substances, such as tobacco smoke, radon, and certain chemicals used in the workplace, can increase your risk of developing cancer. Taking steps to limit your exposure to these substances is important for cancer prevention.

Get Vaccinated: Some cancers, such as cervical cancer, can be prevented by getting vaccinated against the virus that causes them. Talk to your doctor about which vaccines you may need to reduce your risk of developing cancer.

Maintain a Healthy Weight: Being overweight or obese can increase your risk of developing several types of cancer, including breast, colorectal, and endometrial cancer. Maintaining a healthy weight through diet and exercise can help reduce your risk of developing cancer.

Remember, the best way to prevent cancer is to take a comprehensive approach that includes healthy lifestyle habits, regular screening, and avoidance of harmful substances. Talk to your doctor about what you can do to reduce your risk of developing cancer and to catch it early if it does occur.

A. Lifestyle Changes for Cancer Prevention

How may one lessen their risk of developing cancer? Plenty of guidance is available. But sometimes, recommendations from one research conflict with those from another.

Information on cancer prevention is always evolving. But it's well acknowledged that a person's lifestyle might influence their risk of developing cancer.

To avoid cancer, take into account these lifestyle recommendations.

1. Give up smoking

Numerous cancers, including those of the lung, mouth, throat, voice box, pancreas, bladder, cervix, and kidney, have been associated with smoking. The chance of developing lung cancer may even rise when secondhand smoking is present.

But dangerous behaviors are not limited to smoking. The mouth, throat, and pancreas have all been related to tobacco use via chewing.

Avoiding tobacco use or resolving to quit using it is a crucial step in cancer prevention. Ask your doctor about stop-smoking aids and other methods of stopping if you need assistance.

2. Consume a balanced diet

Though it cannot guarantee cancer prevention, consuming healthful meals may lower the risk. Think about the following:

Consume a lot of fruits and veggies. Focus on eating fruits, vegetables, and other plant-based foods as the foundation of your diet, such as whole grains and legumes. Choosing fewer high-calorie items can help you eat lighter and leaner. Limit your intake of processed carbohydrates and animal-sourced fat.
If you do consume alcohol, do it in moderation. Cancer of the breast, colon, lungs, kidneys, and liver are just a few of the cancers that are made more likely by alcohol. Increased consumption raises the danger.
Eat less processed meat. Consuming processed meat often may marginally raise your chance of developing several cancers. This information was found in a report from the World Health Organization's International Agency for Research on Cancer.
Breast cancer risk may be decreased in those who follow a Mediterranean diet that includes

extra-virgin olive oil and mixed nuts. The mainstays of the Mediterranean diet include plant-based foods such fruits, vegetables, whole grains, legumes, and nuts. Olive oil is preferred over butter by those who consume a Mediterranean diet. Red meat isn't eaten there; fish is.

3. Keep a healthy weight and engage in physical activity.
Some cancers may be less likely to develop in people who are in a healthy weight range. Breast, prostate, lung, colon, and kidney cancer are among them.

Exercise is also taken into account. Physical exercise on its own may reduce the incidence of breast cancer and colon cancer in addition to aiding with weight management.

Any physical exercise is good for your health. However, aim for at least 150 minutes of moderate aerobic exercise or 75 minutes of vigorous aerobic activity each week for the most effect.

You can engage in both strenuous and gentle exercise. Include at least 30 minutes of physical exercise each day as a general objective. Better is more.

4. Avoid exposure to the sun.
One of the most prevalent and most curable forms of cancer is skin cancer. Try the following advice:

Skip the noon sun. When the sun's rays are at their fiercest, between 10 a.m. and 4 p.m., stay out of the sun.
Keep to the shadows. When outside, try to spend as much time in the shade as you can. Additionally helpful are a wide-brimmed hat and sunglasses.
Shield your skin. Wear clothes that completely encloses your body. Wear sunglasses and a head covering. Wear striking or dark hues. They

reflect more of the sun's damaging rays than pastels or cotton that has been bleached.

Don't cut corners on sunscreen. Even on overcast days, use a broad-spectrum sunscreen with an SPF of at least 30. Make liberal use of sunscreen. After swimming or perspiring, reapply more often than every two hours.

Avoid using sunlamps or tanning beds. These provide as equal risk of injury as sunshine.

5. Obtain a vaccine.

Defending against certain viral infections may aid in cancer prevention. Consult a medical professional about becoming immunized against:

B-type hepatitis Liver cancer risk may rise as a result of hepatitis B. Adults who have sex with several partners, one sexual partner who has sex with multiple partners, and those who have STDs are at a greater risk of contracting hepatitis B.

People who inject illicit substances, males who have intercourse with other men, and public safety or healthcare employees who could come into touch with contaminated blood or other fluids are other high-risk groups.

H. papilloma virus (HPV). HPV is a sexually transmitted virus that may cause squamous cell carcinoma of the head and neck in addition to cervical cancer and other genital malignancies. The HPV vaccination is advised for boys and girls between the ages of 11 and 12. Gardasil 9 has just received approval from the U.S. Food and Drug Administration for use in men and females aged 9 to 45.

6. Abstain from dangerous actions

Avoiding dangerous activities that might result in infections, which afterwards may raise the risk of cancer, is another excellent cancer preventive strategy. For instance:

Sex should be safe. Use a condom and limit your sexual partners. The likelihood of contracting an STD like HIV or HPV increases with the number of sexual partners one has over the course of a lifetime.

Cancers of the lung, anus, and liver are more common in those with HIV or AIDS. The anus, penis, throat, vulva, and vaginal cancers may all be at increased risk as a result of HPV, which is most often linked to cervical cancer.

Never exchange needles. Sharing needles while injecting drugs increases the chance of contracting hepatitis B and C, which may raise the risk of liver cancer. Consult a specialist if you're worried about drug abuse or addiction.

7. Seek routine medical attention

Regular self-exams and cancer screenings for skin, colon, cervix, and breast cancer may increase the likelihood of discovering cancer early. The likelihood of recovery increases throughout such time. Inquire with a medical professional about your personal cancer screening regimen.

B. The Importance of a Healthy Diet

A healthy diet is essential for overall health, and it can play a significant role in reducing the risk of developing cancer. Research has shown that the foods you eat can impact your body's natural processes and your risk of developing various diseases, including cancer. Here are some of the ways that a healthy diet can help reduce your risk of developing cancer:

1. Antioxidants: Antioxidants are compounds that protect cells from damage caused by free radicals. Fruits and vegetables are rich in antioxidants, and eating a diet high in these foods has been linked to a reduced risk of certain types of cancer, including lung, breast, and prostate cancer.

2. Fiber: Fiber helps to move waste through the digestive system and reduce the amount of time that cancer-causing substances are in contact with the cells of the colon. Whole grains, fruits, and vegetables are good sources of fiber, and a diet high in these foods has been linked to a reduced risk of colon cancer.

3. Lean Protein: Eating a diet high in lean protein, such as fish, poultry, and legumes, has been linked to a reduced risk of certain types of cancer. These foods are lower in fat and calories than red meat and are also good sources of important nutrients like iron and B vitamins.

4. Limit Processed and Red Meat: Processed and red meat have been linked to an increased risk of certain types of cancer, including colon, breast, and prostate cancer. Limiting your consumption of these foods and choosing lean proteins instead can help reduce your risk of developing these cancers.

5. Avoid Added Sugars: Added sugars are found in many processed foods, snacks, and drinks and have been linked to an increased risk of certain types of cancer, including endometrial and breast cancer. Limiting your consumption of added sugars and choosing whole, minimally processed foods instead can help reduce your risk of developing cancer.

In addition to a healthy diet, maintaining a healthy weight, getting regular physical activity, and avoiding exposure to harmful substances can also help reduce your risk of developing cancer. It's important to talk to your doctor about what you can do to support your overall health and reduce your risk of developing cancer.

C. Exercise and Physical Activity

Exercise and physical activity are important for overall health and can play a significant role in reducing the risk of developing cancer. Regular physical activity has been linked to a reduced risk of several types of cancer, including breast, colon, endometrial, and lung cancer.

There are several types of exercise and physical activity that can be beneficial for cancer treatment and prevention. ***Here are some of the most effective types:***

Aerobic Exercise: Aerobic exercise, also known as cardio, can help improve cardiovascular health, boost immune function, and reduce the risk of developing several types of cancer. Examples of aerobic exercise include running, cycling, and swimming.

Resistance Training: Resistance training, also known as strength training, can help build muscle mass and improve bone density. This type of exercise has been linked to a reduced risk of breast, prostate, and colon cancer.

Yoga: Yoga is a form of physical and mental exercise that can help reduce stress, improve flexibility, and increase strength. Some studies have suggested that yoga may also help reduce the risk of breast and colon cancer.

HIIT is a form of exercise that involves short bursts of high-intensity activity followed by periods of rest. HIIT has been shown to improve cardiovascular health, boost insulin sensitivity, and reduce the risk of several types of cancer.

Tai Chi: Tai Chi is a low-impact form of exercise that involves slow, controlled movements and deep breathing. Tai Chi has been linked to improved balance and reduced stress, and some studies have suggested that it may also help reduce the risk of breast and prostate cancer.

It's important to remember that the best type of exercise for cancer treatment and prevention will depend on several factors, including overall health, age, and fitness level. It's recommended that individuals speak with their doctor before starting a new exercise routine to ensure it's safe and appropriate for their needs.

Here are some of the ways that exercise and physical activity can help reduce your risk of developing cancer:

Maintains a Healthy Weight: Regular exercise can help maintain a healthy weight, and obesity is a risk factor for several types of cancer, including breast, colon, endometrial, and kidney cancer.

Reduces Inflammation: Physical activity can reduce inflammation in the body, and chronic inflammation has been linked to an increased risk of several types of cancer, including colorectal, breast, and prostate cancer.

Boosts Immune Function: Exercise has been shown to boost immune function, and a healthy immune system is important for fighting off cancer and other diseases.

Improves Insulin Sensitivity: Regular physical activity has been shown to improve insulin sensitivity, and insulin resistance is a risk factor for several types of cancer, including endometrial and breast cancer.

Reduces Exposure to Harmful Substances: Exercise can help reduce the amount of time that cancer-causing substances are in contact with the cells of the colon, and physical activity has also been linked to a reduced risk of lung cancer by reducing exposure to harmful substances in the air.

Exercise seems to significantly reduce the incidence of the following seven cancers: bladder, breast, colon, endometrial, esophageal, kidney, and stomach. There are also fascinating hints that suggest exercise lowers the risk of malignancies of the head and neck, pancreas, ovary, lung, and prostate.

All cancer patients are highly advised to stay active and engage in regular exercise.

Cancer patients may safely exercise provided it is properly prescribed and monitored. Cancer patients with complicated or uncontrolled diseases often need to take precautions. As a result, some individuals would need a modified program, while others could need to put off beginning a program.

Before beginning an exercise program, consult with a certified health expert (such as your cancer specialists, GP, exercise physiologist, or physiotherapist) if you have any concerns about its safety.

If you suffer from any of the following ailments, you may need to modify your workout routine:

1. pain
2. Lymphedema
3. mild to severe exhaustion
4. anemia
5. pronounced breathlessness 6. a low platelet count
7. Burns after radiation treatment

8. impaired immune system; 9. nerve damage (peripheral neuropathy)
10. Bone cancer, either primary or metastatic.

If you have severe anemia, fever, or extreme weight loss, you should postpone starting an activity program.

It's crucial to make an effort to be active physically. While some days may be more difficult than others, any amount of mild activity is preferable than none at all.

advantages of exercise for cancer patients
Although exercise is excellent for us all, evidence shows that it is especially beneficial in the treatment of cancer. In fact, research indicates that one of the finest things cancer patients can do in addition to their cancer treatment regimen is exercise.

That's because cancer treatment side effects are less and less frequent in persons who exercise frequently. Those who become more active after receiving a cancer diagnosis may also have a decreased risk of both cancer death and cancer recurrence.

The advantages of exercise for cancer patients may include:

i. better health and happiness
enhanced athletic prowess, muscular power, and endurance
ii. more vigor and less weariness caused by cancer
iii. increased mood and a reduction in stress, despair, and anxiety
iv. enhanced heart health and a lower chance of developing heart disease
enhanced flexibility and joint range of motion
better bone density and decreased risk of osteoporosis

v. greater balance and less chance of falling; decreased nausea and vomiting for certain chemotherapy patients; better appetite; deeper, more restorative sleep; improved digestion;

decreased constipation; increased sensations of control over your life.

These advantages may speed up your recovery and lessen treatment-related adverse effects including tiredness, anxiety, sadness, and muscular weakness. Exercise and a balanced diet may help you live a healthy, active lifestyle and help you get back into work, everyday life, and relationships with friends, family, and coworkers.

Before beginning a fitness regimen while fighting cancer
It's crucial to discuss any necessary precautions with a qualified healthcare provider before beginning any fitness regimen, whether it is during or after your treatment. This includes your oncologist, general practitioner, a physiotherapist or exercise physiologist with knowledge in treating cancer patients, among others.

Start softly and increase your activity level gradually if it has been a while since you last exercised or if your fitness level is poor. It's crucial to pay attention to your body. While effort is necessary for exercise, you don't want to push yourself so hard that you experience pain or significant discomfort.

It might be intimidating to begin a fitness routine. Considering that everyone is affected by illness and therapy in a different way, seeing an exercise physiologist may be extremely beneficial. These university-educated health experts have the expertise and talents to provide you a specially designed fitness regimen based on your abilities and present condition.

D. Avoiding Cancer-Causing Substances

The chance of acquiring cancer may be decreased in large part by avoiding cancer-causing chemicals. Tobacco, alcohol, and exposure to dangerous chemicals and pollutants are a few of the most often occurring cancer-causing factors.

Tobacco: Tobacco is the world's largest cause of fatalities that might have been prevented and accounts for around 30% of all cancer deaths. Tar and carbon monoxide, two of the more than 70 cancer-causing compounds found in tobacco, may harm DNA and raise the chance of getting cancer. One of the best methods to lower your chances of developing cancer is to stop smoking or using tobacco products.

Alcohol: Drinking alcohol is known to increase the chance of developing numerous cancers, including breast, liver, and colorectal cancer. Alcohol is thought to be metabolized into hazardous substances that may harm DNA and other biological components, however the precise process by which alcohol raises the risk of cancer is not fully known. Reducing alcohol intake is a crucial first step in lowering the risk of cancer.

Exposure to Dangerous Chemicals and Pollutants: Cancer risk may also be increased by exposure to dangerous chemicals and pollutants. This covers being exposed to chemicals at work as well as pollution from the environment, such as air and water pollution. Cancer risk may be decreased by limiting exposure to certain drugs.

A healthy lifestyle, which includes eating a balanced diet, exercising often, and controlling stress, is crucial in addition to avoiding cancer-causing drugs. These routines may strengthen the immune system and lower the chance of cancer development.

Proactive cancer screening and early diagnosis are also crucial. Mammograms and colonoscopies are two common cancer screening procedures that may help find cancer early, when therapy is more likely to be effective.

In conclusion, minimizing the risk of cancer begins with avoiding drugs that cause it. It's important to be aware of the chemicals to which we are exposed and to take action to minimize exposure wherever possible. A healthy lifestyle, routine cancer screenings, and aggressive early detection strategies may all help lower the risk of cancer and enhance general health.

E. Cancer Screening and Early Detection

Critical elements of cancer prevention and therapy include cancer screening and early detection. Early diagnosis enables early treatment, increasing the likelihood of a favorable result.

Cancer screenings come in a variety of forms, including blood testing, imaging studies, and physical examinations. Mammograms for breast cancer, colonoscopies for gastrointestinal cancer, and PSA testing for prostate cancer are a few examples of frequent cancer screenings.

The ability to detect cancer early on, before symptoms appear, is one of the main advantages of cancer screening. When the cancer is more curable and has not had a time to spread to other places of the body, this enables quicker treatment. Early identification may boost the possibility of a full recovery and favorable treatment outcomes.

The ability to identify cancer in high-risk patients before symptoms appear is a significant advantage of cancer screening. This includes those with a history of cancer in their families as well as those who have additional risk factors such advanced age, certain lifestyle choices, and exposure to carcinogens.

The purpose of cancer screening and early detection is to prevent cancer by identifying malignancies or their precursor lesions before symptoms appear, when cancer therapy is most successful. In fact, total cancer mortality in the United States declined by 25% between 1990 and 2015, with even higher drops in colorectal cancer mortality (47% among men and 44% among women) and breast cancer mortality (39% among women). The emergence of high-quality colorectal and breast cancer screening may be partly blamed for this decline.

The most effective cancer screening programs identify precursor lesions (e.g., colonic polyps with colorectal cancer screening and cervical intraepithelial neoplasia (CIN) with cervical cancer screening), which are then treated to reduce the incidence of invasive cancer over time.

Wilson and Jungner of the World Health Organization put forward the fundamental principles for illness screening in 1968. Not all suggestions for cancer screening adhere to all of these guiding principles; traditionally, a compromise has been struck between the detection of early or precursor lesions and the prevention of overdiagnosis, which might result in overtreatment.

In conclusion, early cancer identification and screening are essential to the prevention and management of cancer. Cancer screening may considerably increase the likelihood of a favorable result by detecting cancer in its earlier stages, when therapy is more likely to be effective. It's crucial to go through the recommended routine cancer screenings and discuss your own risk factors and screening choices with your healthcare professional.

Chapter 3

The Anti-Cancer Mindset

The anti-cancer mindset is a critical component of cancer treatment and recovery. This mindset is about embracing a positive outlook, focusing on the present moment, and taking an active role in one's own healing journey.

A. Positive Thinking and Mindfulness

Positive thinking and mindfulness are important tools in developing an anti-cancer mindset. By focusing on positive thoughts and emotions, individuals can reduce stress, improve mood, and increase their sense of control over their lives. Mindfulness practices, such as meditation and deep breathing, can help individuals stay centered and focused, even in the face of challenges.

Mindfulness, on the other hand, is the practice of being fully present in the moment, without judgment or distraction. It involves paying attention to one's thoughts, feelings, and physical sensations, and accepting them without trying to change them. Mindfulness has been shown to be effective in reducing stress, anxiety, and depression, and in improving well-being.

Positive thinking and mindfulness are interrelated and complement each other in promoting a healthy anti-cancer mindset. Positive thinking can help individuals maintain hope and optimism, while mindfulness can help individuals stay centered and focused, even in the face of challenges.

To develop positive thinking and mindfulness, individuals can engage in a variety of practices, such as:

Gratitude: Taking time to reflect on the things in life that one is thankful for, and expressing gratitude for them.

Affirmations: Repeating positive self-statements, such as "I am strong and capable," to reinforce positive thinking and increase self-confidence.

Visualization: Imagining a positive outcome or future, such as successfully completing cancer treatment or being cancer-free, to maintain hope and optimism.

Mindfulness meditation: Sitting quietly and focusing on the present moment, without judgment or distraction, to reduce stress and increase well-being.

Deep breathing: Taking slow, deep breaths to calm the mind and reduce stress.

Incorporating positive thinking and mindfulness into daily life can help individuals maintain hope and optimism, reduce stress, and improve well-being, all of which are important components of the anti-cancer mindset. By embracing these practices, individuals can take an active role in their own healing journey and increase their chances of a successful outcome.

B. Coping with a Cancer Diagnosis

Receiving a cancer diagnosis can be a shock and a source of stress, but it's important to remember that it's possible to cope and even thrive in the face of this challenge. By developing a strong support network, learning about the disease, and engaging in self-care practices such as exercise, individuals can gain a sense of control and maintain hope and optimism.

It might be challenging to learn that you have cancer. Some claim that when they were first diagnosed, they had feelings of anxiety, fear, or overwhelm. Here are 11 suggestions to assist you cope with a cancer diagnosis if you are unsure of how to proceed.

1. Find out the details of your cancer diagnosis. Get as much valuable understanding as you can. This will support your decision-making on your care.

Make a list of your inquiries and worries. When you want to see your doctor, bring them with you.

2. You may question:

i. the kind of cancer I have?
ii. Cancer is present where?
iii. Has it grown?
iv. Is there a cure for my cancer?
v. What are the chances of curing my cancer?
vi. What more exams or treatments are required?
vii. What alternatives do I have for treatment?
viii. How will the medication help me?
ix. What should I anticipate from my treatment?
x. What adverse effects might the medicine cause?
xi. When should I make a call to my doctor?
xii. What can I do to stop the cancer from returning?

xiii. How probable is it that my kids or other family members may get cancer?
xiv. What will occur if I don't get treatment?

At least one family member or close friend should accompany you to your first visits. They may aid in retaining what you hear.

3. Consider how much information you want to have about your cancer. Some folks want complete information. They may participate in decision-making because of this. Others choose to get a basic understanding and leave specifics and choices up to their healthcare professionals. Consider which option suits you the best. Tell the medical staff what you would want.

Maintain open channels of communication
Maintain open lines of communication with those you love, medical professionals, and others. If others attempt to shield you from terrible news by not talking about it, you could feel alone. If you strive to seem tough and hide your emotions, you could also feel alone or less

supported. You may assist one another if you both express your true sentiments.

Be prepared for any physical changes
The optimum time to make plans for physical changes is soon after receiving a cancer diagnosis and before you start treatment. Make your preparations now so that you can handle everything afterwards.

What may change? Inquire with your healthcare practitioner. Losing your hair may be caused by medications. You may feel more at ease and appealing with the support of professional advice on your appearance in terms of clothes, cosmetics, wigs, and hairpieces. Wigs and other adaptation aids are often covered by insurance.

Join a cancer support group if you're interested. Members may share advice that has benefited both themselves and others.

Consider how your everyday life will be affected by the therapy as well. Find out from your provider whether you can go on with your regular schedule. You may have to stay in the hospital for a while or attend a lot of doctor's visits. Make plans for this if your treatment will make it difficult for you to carry out your regular responsibilities.

Prepare your funds in advance. Decide who will do the usual home tasks. Please ask someone to look after your pets if you have any.

4. Keep up a fit lifestyle
Your energy level might increase with a healthy lifestyle. Pick a balanced diet. Take time to relax. This advice can aid you in controlling the stress and exhaustion associated with cancer and its treatment.

Have a steady daily schedule if you can. Make sure to schedule time each day for eating, sleeping, and exercising.

Exercise and engaging in enjoyable hobbies may both be beneficial. Exercise during therapy helps patients manage side effects better and may even extend their lives.

Let relatives and friends assist you.
Your friends and family can assist you with errands, transportation to appointments, food preparation, and housework. This might provide your loved ones a method to support you through a difficult period.

Encourage your family to accept assistance if it is required. The whole family is impacted by a cancer diagnosis. It also causes stress, particularly for those who are responsible for your care. Receiving assistance from friends or neighbors with housework or meals helps prevent your loved ones from being overworked.

5. Review your priorities and ambitions.
Determine what matters most to you in life. Make time for the things that are most meaningful to you and are most essential to you. Examine your schedule and cancel any appointments that don't fit your objectives.

6. With your loved ones, try to be honest.
Tell them your emotions and opinions. All of your relationships are impacted by cancer. Cancer-related anxiety and worry may be lessened through communication.

7. Try to keep up your way of life.
Keep your way of life, but be willing to adapt to it. Take each day as it comes. It's simple to forget to do this while under pressure. Planning and arranging may suddenly seem like too much labor when the future is uncertain.

8. Think about the financial effect of your diagnosis.
After receiving a cancer diagnosis, many unforeseen financial problems may arise. Time away from home or work may be necessary for your therapy. Take into account the price of prescription drugs, medical equipment, travel expenses for treatment, and hospital parking fees.

To assist you financially during and after your cancer treatment, several clinics and hospitals maintain lists of resources. Discuss your alternatives with your medical team.

9. Ones to consider asking are:

1. Will I have to miss any work time? What will happen to my benefits if I do that?
2. Will my relatives and friends have to skip work so they can be with me?
3. Will these therapies be covered by my insurance?
4. Will the price of medications be covered by my insurance? What will the price be?
5. Exist any services that can assist me if my insurer refuses to cover my care?
6. Can I get disability benefits?
7. What impact will my diagnosis have on my life insurance?
8. To find out what my insurance will cover, who should I contact?

10.Talk to other cancer sufferers.

People who have not had cancer may find it difficult to comprehend how you feel. Speaking with others who have experienced your circumstance might be helpful. You may hear from other cancer survivors about their stories. They can explain what to anticipate from the process of therapy.

Speak with a friend or relative who has battled cancer. Or join a support group to communicate with other cancer survivors. Inquire with your healthcare practitioner about local support groups. You may get in touch with your neighborhood American Cancer Society branch. Online message boards also bring cancer survivors together. Start with the Cancer Survivors Network of the American Cancer Society.

Speak with friends or neighbors who have just recovered from a terrible illness. Ask them how they resolved these challenging problems.

11. Combat stigmas

There are certain persistent cancer stigmas. Your pals may query if your cancer is communicable. Coworkers could question if you're fit enough to do your duties. Some people may avoid you out of a fear of saying anything inappropriate. There will be plenty of queries and worries.

Decide how you'll interact with other people. In general, others will copy your actions. Remind friends that they shouldn't be frightened to be near you because of your disease.

Create your own strategies for combating cancer. The methods used to treat cancer vary depending on the patient, much as their cancer therapy does. Tips to consider

12. Train yourself to relax.

Honestly express your emotions to loved ones, friends, a spiritual leader, or a counselor.
To help you arrange your ideas, keep a diary.

When presented with a tough choice, make a list of the advantages and disadvantages of each option.

Look for a spiritual resource to help you.

Make time for solitude.

Maintain as much involvement in your job and leisure pursuits as you can.

Be prepared to refuse. Take a moment to think about yourself.

What got you through difficult moments before your cancer diagnosis may be able to aid you today. This might be a personal companion, a spiritual figure, or a pastime. Now rely on this consolation. Be willing to test novel cancer treatments as well.

C. Maintaining Hope and Optimism

A critical component of cancer therapy and recovery is maintaining optimism and hope. Although the trip may be arduous and demanding, maintaining a positive mindset may significantly affect both the mental and emotional components of the experience.

The capacity of the body to fight cancer may be improved, which is one of the primary advantages of keeping hope and optimism. According to research, thinking positively and having a cheerful attitude may strengthen the immune system, give people more energy, and lessen stress and worry. In turn, this may enhance the patient's general health and wellbeing and raise their chances of having a positive result.

Maintaining optimism and hope has the added advantage of enhancing the patient's quality of life. Maintaining a positive perspective may assist to lower stress and anxiety as well as enhance general mood and well-being throughout cancer treatment, which can be both physically and emotionally taxing.

It's crucial to keep in mind that retaining optimism and hope is a subjective experience.

Finding what works best for you is crucial since what works for one person may not work for another. This might include doing things that make you happy and joyful, getting in touch with encouraging friends and family members, and getting help from a mental health expert.

Here are some of the top tips discovered for maintaining optimism while receiving cancer treatment:

1.Your best ally is you. Nobody is more concerned about your health than you are. You have to take charge. If you are wallowing in self-pity and negativity, you cannot do that. Maintain a good attitude and surround yourself with enthusiastic, positive individuals.

2. Keep thorough notes. Every discussion from every test, meeting, and phone call should be documented. Your memory is impacted since chemo-brain is a really genuine condition. To take notes, a simple spiral notebook will do. Keep good records so that others may assist you and you can make better judgments. We have gone back to my notes so many times that I can't even count.

3. Pay attention to the factors in your control. I have no idea when or if I will ever stop taking the clinical trial medications, or whether we will always make a monthly trip to Houston. But I make an effort to ignore it. I've discovered that concentrating on the areas I can control, like my eating habits, is considerably more useful. I now make every effort to stay away from processed foods, chemicals, and preservatives, and my husband and I have all but eliminated sugar from our diets.

4. Don't limit the talk to health-related issues. No matter how close you are to your pals, I assure you that they don't want to hear you go on about your most recent treatments, complaints about physicians and hospitals, etc. If they inquire how you are, give a brief summary, say "fine," and then thank them before leaving. Stay upbeat.

5. Be grateful for your family. Love your partner and the people who are taking care of you, and be as optimistic as you can. They are likewise experiencing suffering and agony. Each and every visit, infusion, and the majority of the biopsies have been accompanied by my loving spouse. We sometimes had to nag the biopsy room staff to let him in. He has been and still is my pillar of support. I try to keep in mind to give him frequent thanks for what he has done for me.

6. Establish a strong network of allies. Speak to your doctor or insurance provider if you don't have any relatives or friends who can serve as a support system. Make every effort to surround yourself with upbeat, encouraging individuals who will encourage you, get you out of the home, and divert your attention from your troubles.

7. Keep trying. I am aware that nothing is certain, particularly with cancer. But developments are happening more quickly than ever before, so resist the urge to give up and cower in a corner. Because I refused to just accept the treatment I was receiving, I am still here today. My husband and I took the initiative and looked for something we believed in when we were unsatisfied with the therapy alternatives available at home, such as this clinical study at MD Anderson. I am immediately reminded of how grateful I am that I didn't give up hope when I consider all the things I would have missed if I had just withdrawn from society and my family. I really hope you never do the same.

In conclusion, a critical component of cancer therapy and recovery is keeping hope and optimism. Keeping a positive mindset may significantly influence the overall outcome of therapy by enhancing the body's capacity to fight cancer and boosting quality of life in general. As you traverse this difficult road, it's crucial to identify what works best for you and ask for help from people around you.

D. The Role of Support Systems

It is impossible to overestimate the importance of support systems throughout the course of cancer treatment and recovery. When it comes to assisting people in navigating the physical, emotional, and practical obstacles that come with a cancer diagnosis, having a solid support system in place may make all the difference.

The ability to get emotional assistance is one of the main advantages of having a support system. Having people in your life who get what you are going through and can provide comfort and support may be crucial since dealing with cancer can be a stressful and daunting journey. This may be done with the help of friends, family, support groups, or even a mental health specialist.

Practical assistance is a key component of support systems. Having someone in your life who can assist with things like transportation to and from appointments, food shopping, or child care may have a major influence on overall well-being. Cancer treatment can be physically and emotionally taxing.

As different people may provide various sorts of support, it is crucial to have a range of support networks in place. A close friend, for instance, may give emotional support, whilst a family member would offer practical help. A network of dependable people may help lower stress and anxiety and enhance general quality of life.

In addition to having established support systems, it's critical to actively seek out and make use of such systems. This may include contacting friends and relatives, joining a support group, or looking for a mental health expert's advice.

Chapter 4

Integrative Cancer Treatment

Integrative cancer treatment refers to the combination of traditional cancer treatments with complementary and alternative therapies to improve overall health and well-being during and after treatment. This approach recognizes that cancer is a complex disease and that a variety of treatments may be necessary to achieve the best possible outcomes.

A. Traditional Cancer Treatments

Traditional Cancer Treatments refer to the standard medical treatments for cancer that have been widely used and accepted as effective in treating cancer. These treatments are based on extensive research and clinical trials, and have been proven to be effective in many cases.

The main types of traditional cancer treatments include:

Surgery: This is a procedure to remove the cancerous tissue. It may involve removing the entire tumor or only a portion of it. Surgery can be performed to cure the cancer, to relieve symptoms, or to diagnose the disease.

Radiation therapy: This is a treatment that uses high-energy radiation to kill cancer cells. Radiation can be delivered externally, from a machine outside the body, or internally, from radioactive material placed inside the body.

Chemotherapy: This is a treatment that uses drugs to kill cancer cells. Chemotherapy can be given orally, by injection, or intravenously. It may be given alone or in combination with other treatments, such as surgery or radiation therapy.

Hormonal therapy: This is a treatment that manipulates the levels of hormones in the body to stop the growth of certain types of cancers, such as breast and prostate cancer. Hormonal therapy may involve taking drugs that block the production of hormones or interfere with their action.

Targeted therapy: This is a type of treatment that targets specific molecules in cancer cells that allow them to grow and divide. Targeted therapy can be used in combination with other treatments, such as chemotherapy or radiation therapy, to improve outcomes and reduce side effects.

Immunotherapy: This is a type of treatment that uses the body's immune system to fight cancer. It may involve using drugs to boost the immune system's response to cancer, or to remove obstacles that prevent the immune system from recognizing and destroying cancer cells.

Stem cell transplant: This is a procedure in which healthy stem cells are transplanted into the body to replace damaged or destroyed cells, including blood-forming stem cells that have been damaged by chemotherapy or radiation therapy.

Hyperthermia: This is a type of treatment that uses heat to destroy cancer cells. It may be delivered externally, using a machine to apply heat to the tumor, or internally, using a special probe that delivers heat directly to the cancer.

Photodynamic therapy (PDT): This is a type of treatment that uses light and a special drug called a photosensitizer to kill cancer cells. The photosensitizer is given to the patient and then exposed to a special light, which activates the drug and destroys the cancer cells.

Proton therapy: This is a type of radiation therapy that uses protons, rather than x-rays, to treat cancer. Proton therapy is considered more precise and effective than traditional x-ray radiation, as it delivers higher doses of radiation to the tumor while minimizing exposure to surrounding healthy tissue.

These treatments are designed to target and destroy cancer cells, while minimizing harm to healthy cells. The choice of treatment depends on many factors, including the type of cancer, the stage of the cancer, and the overall health of the patient. Traditional cancer treatments can be effective in treating cancer, but they can also cause significant side effects and stress to the body.

B. Complementary and Alternative Therapies

Complementary and alternative therapies (CAM) are non-traditional approaches to cancer treatment that may be used alongside conventional treatments like surgery, chemotherapy, and radiation therapy. These therapies are designed to help manage symptoms, improve quality of life, and support the body's natural healing processes.

Here are some of the most commonly used complementary and alternative therapies for cancer:

Acupuncture: This is a traditional Chinese therapy that involves the insertion of thin needles into specific points on the body to balance energy flow and promote healing. It may be used to relieve pain, improve sleep, and boost the immune system.

Massage therapy: Massage therapy can help relieve stress, anxiety, and pain and improve sleep and immune function. It may also be used to help manage side effects from conventional treatments like chemotherapy-induced nausea and fatigue.

Mind-body techniques: This group of therapies includes meditation, yoga, and visualization, and is designed to help individuals manage stress, improve their mental health, and boost their overall sense of well-being.

Nutritional therapy: A healthy diet can play a critical role in the treatment and management of cancer. Nutritional therapy can help individuals maintain optimal health and improve their overall quality of life by incorporating foods that support the body's natural healing processes and avoiding those that may promote the growth of cancer cells.

Herbal medicine: Herbs and plant-based remedies have been used for centuries to treat a variety of health conditions, including cancer. Some herbs and supplements may have anti-cancer properties and may be used to support the body's natural healing processes or to manage side effects from conventional treatments.

It is important to note that not all complementary and alternative therapies have been scientifically proven to be safe and effective, and some may interact with conventional treatments. It is important to discuss the use of complementary and alternative therapies with your doctor to determine what is best for your individual needs and health status.

C. The Importance of a Multidisciplinary Approach

In cancer treatment, a multidisciplinary approach refers to a team of healthcare professionals from different specialties working together to develop a comprehensive treatment plan for a patient. This approach is considered to be the most effective way to treat cancer because it leverages the expertise of multiple specialists, resulting in a more holistic and individualized approach to treatment.

A multidisciplinary team typically includes oncologists, radiation therapists, surgeons, nurses, dietitians, and other specialists. This team of experts works together to evaluate a patient's health, determine the best course of action, and develop a treatment plan that meets their specific needs.

One of the key benefits of a multidisciplinary approach is that it provides patients with a more comprehensive understanding of their condition and treatment options. This includes an evaluation of their overall health, the stage and type of cancer they have, and the risks and benefits of different treatment options. With this information, patients are better equipped to make informed decisions about their treatment and to manage the physical, emotional, and social impacts of cancer.

Another advantage of a multidisciplinary approach is that it facilitates coordinated care, ensuring that patients receive the best possible treatment for their particular type and stage of cancer. This includes regular follow-up appointments, monitoring for side effects, and referrals to other specialists as needed.

Overall, a multidisciplinary approach is considered to be the best way to treat cancer because it combines the expertise of multiple specialists, provides patients with a comprehensive understanding of their condition and treatment options, and facilitates coordinated care. By working together, a multidisciplinary team can help patients achieve the best possible outcomes, both in terms of their health and their quality of life.

D. Making an Informed Decision About Treatment

When it comes to cancer treatment, the most important decision a patient can make is the choice of treatment they receive. This decision can have a significant impact on their health, quality of life, and overall outcome. That's why it is crucial for patients to make an informed decision about their treatment, one that is based on a thorough understanding of their condition, the treatment options available, and the potential benefits and risks of each.

One of the first steps in making an informed decision about treatment is to work with a multidisciplinary team of healthcare professionals, as discussed in the previous section. This team can provide a comprehensive evaluation of a patient's health, including the stage and type of cancer they have, and help them understand the different treatment options available.

It is also important for patients to educate themselves about their condition and the various treatment options available. This can involve reading up on the latest research and treatments, talking to other patients and their families, and seeking the advice of healthcare professionals.

Ultimately, the decision about treatment should be made in consultation with a patient's healthcare team and should take into account the patient's individual needs, values, and preferences. For example, some patients may prioritize preserving their quality of life, while others may be more concerned with the potential side effects of treatment.

Making an informed decision about treatment is a personal and deeply important choice, and it is essential for patients to take the time to understand their options and make a decision that is right for them. By doing so, they can increase their chances of a positive outcome, both in terms of their health and their quality of life.

Chapter 5

Escaping statistics

When it comes to cancer, statistics can be overwhelming and sometimes even discouraging. While it's important to have a general understanding of the disease, it's equally important to remember that statistics should not dictate one's approach to treatment and prevention. Each person's experience with cancer is unique and the statistics that apply to a larger population may not necessarily apply to an individual case.

For example, it's commonly known that the survival rate for a certain type of cancer may be low, but it's important to understand that the survival rate is not always an accurate predictor of an individual's outcome. Factors such as age, overall health, stage of cancer, and the type of treatment received can greatly impact a person's prognosis.

Additionally, it's also important to be cautious about the sources of information used to gather cancer statistics. Data may come from outdated sources or may not take into account new advancements in cancer research and treatments.

In conclusion, while statistics can provide some general insights into the prevalence and outcomes of cancer, it's important to remember that they do not determine an individual's experience with the disease. It's always best to seek out up-to-date, trustworthy information and consult with a medical professional for a personalized approach to cancer treatment and prevention.

Managing uncertainty
I. Express your feelings.
ii. Take a more active role in your own treatment.
iii. heed the counsel of your cancer team.
I'll pay attention to your health.

v. recognize when you need assistance with overwhelming emotions and where to obtain it.

10 techniques to boost self-esteem

It may be difficult and typically requires time and work to increase your sense of self-worth. However, there are certain straightforward actions you may do each day to boost your self-esteem.

1. Highlight the little victories

Positive thinking may help us overcome negative thought patterns and lift our spirits. At the conclusion of each day, try writing down a few encouraging things. Consider recent events, a possible action you took, or a praise you were given.

2. Confront a difficulty.

Perhaps you wish to acquire a new skill or return to a past-time passion. Make a doable strategy and give yourself a reasonable deadline. Once you've done that, congratulate yourself and let others do the same.

3. Pay attention more.

We are prone to believing our ideas to be true when we are caught up in them. Thoughts, however, are but that—thoughts—and are not always true. Try adding the words "I'm having the notion that" or saying, "There goes that inner critic again" before damaging thoughts like "I'm rubbish" or "I should be able to deal." These kinds of methods may assist us in taking our ideas less seriously.

4. Have mercy on yourself.

Self-compassion is more about recognizing when we're suffering and not condemning ourselves for it than self-indulgence. If you catch yourself being critical of yourself, ask yourself, "What would I say to a friend?"

5. Look for people who can help.

Embrace the affection and respect of those who are supportive of you. Try the online forums for

Breast Cancer Care or the Someone Like Me service as well.

6. Avoid comparing yourself with others (or yourself before cancer)

We might compare ourselves to our "former self," which is another common comparison trap that we all fall into. Consider all the things you could do before cancer, for instance. We often feel down and self-conscious as a consequence of this. Instead, try to focus on your success thus far and how you can keep moving forward; this will inspire you and boost your self-confidence.

7. Give yourself some time.

We often don't devote enough time to the activities we like or that make us feel good about ourselves. Try to schedule some "me time" each day or each week; don't feel bad about it; you deserve it.

8. Have reasonable expectations.

Give yourself a break! We often blame ourselves when we can't manage or do something because we believe we should be able to. Pace yourself and keep in mind what you've gone through. There is a limit to what is "good enough."

9. Take care of yourself

Eat healthily and work out often. Your mental and physical well-being may both be improved. Exercise may enhance your energy and happiness, and eating healthfully serves as a reminder that you are valuable.

10. Seek assistance if you need it.

Speak to someone about receiving some help if you've tried these suggestions and discovered that they haven't been successful for you. Asking for assistance may be difficult, but your treatment team and doctor will be able to recommend counseling and psychological programs in your area that can support you in exploring these kinds of problems and helping you feel better about yourself.

A. Opportunity and Danger

In the field of cancer treatment, it's important to understand both the opportunities and dangers that come with complementary and alternative therapies. On one hand, these therapies can offer unique and effective approaches to managing the symptoms and side effects of traditional cancer treatments. They can also provide a sense of control and empowerment to individuals who are seeking to actively participate in their own healing journey.

However, it's also important to be cautious when exploring complementary and alternative therapies. Not all of these approaches have been scientifically proven to be safe and effective, and some may even interfere with conventional cancer treatments or harm the body.

It's essential to thoroughly research and understand the potential benefits and risks of each complementary and alternative therapy before making a decision to incorporate it into a cancer treatment plan. It's also recommended to consult with a healthcare professional to ensure that these therapies do not interfere with conventional treatments and to monitor for any potential adverse reactions.

Overall, complementary and alternative therapies can offer opportunities for individuals to take a more proactive role in their cancer treatment journey, but caution must be taken to avoid potential dangers. By educating oneself and working closely with a healthcare team, individuals can make informed decisions about incorporating complementary and alternative therapies into their overall cancer treatment plan.

B. Cancer weakness

In the fight against cancer, it's important to understand the weaknesses of this disease and how they can be exploited to improve treatment outcomes. One of the key weaknesses of cancer is its dependence on blood vessels for growth and survival. Tumors require a constant supply of nutrients and oxygen, which they receive through the development of new blood vessels.

This dependence on blood vessels makes cancer vulnerable to targeted therapies that disrupt the blood supply to the tumor. One example of such a therapy is anti-angiogenic therapy, which blocks the formation of new blood vessels and starves the tumor of the resources it needs to grow and spread.

Another weakness of cancer cells is their instability and susceptibility to DNA damage. This makes them vulnerable to chemotherapy drugs, which target rapidly dividing cells and can cause damage to the DNA of cancer cells, leading to their death.

It's important to note that the weaknesses of cancer cells also present potential opportunities for drug resistance to develop. Cancer cells can adapt and evolve over time, leading to the development of resistance to certain treatments. This highlights the importance of ongoing research and development of new cancer treatments that target the weaknesses of this disease.

By understanding the weaknesses of cancer and exploiting them through targeted therapies and treatments, it becomes possible to improve outcomes and ultimately, find a cure for this devastating disease.

C. Defusing fears

One of the biggest challenges faced by those diagnosed with cancer is overcoming the fear and anxiety that often accompany this diagnosis. This fear can be debilitating and interfere with the ability to make informed decisions about treatment, as well as impact overall quality of life.

However, it's important to understand that many of these fears are often based on misconceptions or incomplete information. Defusing these fears by educating oneself about cancer and the available treatment options can help to reduce anxiety and allow for a clearer and more focused approach to treatment.

One effective way to defuse fears is to seek out credible and reliable sources of information. This could include talking to a healthcare provider, reaching out to support groups, or doing research on reputable websites or organizations.

Another important aspect of defusing fears is to understand the role of hope and optimism in the healing process. Research has shown that a positive outlook and belief in the possibility of recovery can have a significant impact on outcomes, as well as overall well-being.

It's also important to reach out to friends, family, and other support systems for help and comfort. Talking about fears and concerns can help to reduce their intensity and allow for a greater sense of control and empowerment.

How to handle the worry that your cancer may return

Uncertainty is never easy to live with. It's critical to constantly remind oneself that survival is accompanied with feelings of dread and worry. The first year after treatment is often when people worry the most about their cancer returning. In most cases, this anxiety subsides with time; nevertheless, if it persists, you should inform your medical staff.

Here are some suggestions to assist you manage your anxiety of recurrence:

1. Be aware of your feelings. A lot of individuals make an effort to conceal or suppress "bad" emotions like dread and worry. Putting names to them will make it easier for you to come up with solutions.

It often helps to discuss your anxieties with a dependable friend, member of your family, or mental health expert. You may be able to identify the causes of your anxieties by speaking out about them. The dread of needing further cancer treatment, losing control of your life, or passing away are a few examples of this. You may also try maintaining a diary, putting your ideas down, or expressing yourself via music or art.

2. Don't dismiss your worries. It won't help these sensations go away to tell yourself not to worry or to berate yourself for being worried. Recognize that you will feel some dread; then, concentrate on coping mechanisms for the worry. Be aware that your anxiety may spike sometimes at certain periods. For instance, "scanxiety" may strike when you need more imaging scans. The anniversary of your diagnosis, follow-up lab tests or medical appointments, the time when someone else receives a new cancer diagnosis, and other events all often cause this worry to worsen.

You could sometimes worry about scenarios that are unlikely to occur. By addressing the possibility of your issues, talking with your medical team about your concerns might be beneficial.

3. Be a part of a support group. A lot of cancer patients feel that joining a support group is beneficial. The opportunity to express emotions and worries with sympathetic listeners is provided through support groups. You may also provide useful information and constructive advice with them. When survivors participate in groups, they often develop a feeling of belonging that makes them feel less alone and more understood.

4. Select healthful options. People who practice healthy behaviors such as eating wholesome meals, exercising often, and getting adequate sleep feel better physically and mentally. People who abstain from hazardous behaviors like smoking and binge drinking have a greater sense of control over their health. Study up on how to live well after cancer.

5. Lessen tension. Your total level of anxiety will decrease if you can learn to control your stress. To determine what works best for you, try out several stress-reduction techniques.

Tips for lowering stress include:
i. Enjoy time with loved ones and friends.

ii. Concentrate on your interests and other enjoyable pursuits.

iii. Enjoy a stroll, sit in contemplation, or a bath.

iv. Regularly move about.

v. Enjoy a humorous book or television program.

6. Be knowledgeable. Research has been done on the recurrence patterns of various cancer forms. However, nobody can predict with certainty what will occur in the future. The likelihood of the cancer coming back may be discussed with your oncologist or another medical specialist who is familiar with your medical history. They may also provide you with a list of potential symptoms. By being prepared, you may be able to stop worrying that every discomfort indicates the cancer has returned. If you do develop a symptom, discuss it with your medical provider if it persists or worsens.

7. Adhere to your follow-up care schedule. Checking for a cancer recurrence is one of the key objectives of follow-up care. Several weeks, months, or even years after your initial cancer was treated, recurrence might occur. Regular physical exams and/or tests as part of your follow-up treatment plan may be required to monitor your recovery. Having a regular follow-up visit plan might give survivors a feeling of control. Learn more about creating a survivorship care plan.

In conclusion, defusing fears is an important step in the journey towards recovery and improved quality of life for those diagnosed with cancer. By educating oneself, seeking support, and maintaining a positive outlook, it's possible to overcome the fears and anxieties associated with this diagnosis and focus on the path towards recovery.

Chapter 6

The Anti-Cancer Lifestyle

The concept of an "anti-cancer lifestyle" refers to a holistic approach to living that incorporates habits and practices that promote overall health and wellness, and may help to reduce the risk of developing cancer.

At the heart of an anti-cancer lifestyle is the importance of maintaining a healthy diet, engaging in regular exercise and physical activity, avoiding exposure to cancer-causing substances, and maintaining a positive outlook and support system.

Adopting an anti-cancer lifestyle can also involve making other positive changes in one's life, such as quitting smoking, reducing alcohol consumption, reducing stress, and getting regular cancer screenings.

It's important to note that an anti-cancer lifestyle is not a guarantee against developing cancer, but it can help to reduce the risk and improve overall health and well-being. Additionally, incorporating these habits and practices can also have a positive impact on overall quality of life, even if cancer is not a concern.

A. Building a Strong Immune System

Building a strong immune system is crucial in the fight against cancer and maintaining overall health. A strong immune system helps the body identify and destroy abnormal cells, such as cancer cells, before they can cause harm.

There are several factors that contribute to building a strong immune system, including:

1. Eating a balanced and nutritious diet: A diet rich in fruits, vegetables, whole grains, and lean protein provides the nutrients and vitamins necessary for a strong immune system.

2. Regular physical activity: Exercise helps improve circulation, which in turn helps the immune system function more efficiently.

3. Adequate sleep: Getting enough quality sleep is crucial for immune function. Chronic sleep deprivation can weaken the immune system, making it less effective at fighting off infections and diseases.

4. Stress management: Chronic stress has been linked to weakened immune function. Finding effective ways to manage stress, such as mindfulness, exercise, or therapy, can help keep the immune system strong.

5. Avoiding harmful substances: Smoking, excessive alcohol consumption, and exposure to environmental toxins can weaken the immune system.

6. Supplements: Certain supplements, such as vitamins C and D, can help support immune function.

The importance of building a strong immune system cannot be overstated. A strong immune system helps the body fend off infections and diseases, including cancer. Additionally, incorporating habits that support immune function can have a positive impact on overall health and well-being.

B. Maintaining a Healthy Body Weight

Building a powerful immune system and avoiding cancer both depend on maintaining a healthy body weight. Extra body fat has been associated with a higher chance of developing some cancers, including breast, prostate, and colon cancer. Furthermore, being overweight may strain the body's organs and deteriorate the immune system.

A balanced diet full of nutritious foods like fruits, vegetables, lean meats, and whole grains is crucial for maintaining a healthy body weight. Avoiding processed and high-sugar meals may lower the risk of heart disease and type two (2) diabetes as well as assist avoid weight gain.

Another important factor in maintaining a healthy body weight is physical exercise. Regular exercise may assist to increase metabolism, develop muscle, and burn extra body fat. A good example of this would be to work out for 30 minutes most days of the week at a moderate effort. Strength training and aerobic exercise should both be a part of your regimen for extra health advantages including better cardiovascular health and more muscle mass.

Keeping a healthy body weight might include more than just nutrition and exercise. It can also involve controlling your stress levels. Stressful situations might cause hormonal changes that impair immunity and cause overeating and weight gain. By implementing stress-reduction strategies like deep breathing, mindfulness, and exercise into your daily routine, you may promote a strong immune system and maintain a healthy body weight.

C. Getting Enough Sleep

Getting enough sleep is essential for our overall health and well-being, and it is also crucial for those who are trying to prevent or recover from cancer. A good night's sleep helps to restore our bodies, improve our moods, and refresh our minds, allowing us to face each day with energy and enthusiasm. However, for cancer patients, sleep can be more challenging, and getting enough of it can be a critical factor in their recovery.

One of the most important reasons why sleep is so important for cancer patients is because it helps to boost the immune system. During sleep, our bodies produce cytokines, which are essential for fighting off infections and cancer. Additionally, when we are sleeping, our bodies are repairing and regenerating damaged cells, which is crucial for recovery and survival. For this reason, it is vital that cancer patients make sleep a priority, and strive to get at least 7-9 hours of sleep each night.

Unfortunately, many cancer patients struggle with sleep because of the symptoms of the disease and the side effects of treatment. For example, some cancer treatments can cause fatigue, pain, and discomfort, making it difficult to fall asleep or stay asleep. Additionally, many cancer patients experience anxiety, depression, and stress, which can further disrupt sleep patterns.

For cancer patients who are having trouble sleeping, there are a number of strategies that can be helpful. For example, creating a relaxing bedtime routine, such as reading or listening to calming music, can help to prepare the mind and body for sleep. Additionally, practicing relaxation techniques, such as deep breathing or meditation, can help to calm the mind and reduce anxiety.

It is also important for cancer patients to create a sleep-conducive environment, by making sure that the room is cool, dark, and quiet, and that the bed is comfortable. Additionally, avoiding caffeine, nicotine, and alcohol before bedtime can also help to improve sleep quality.

D. Managing Stress

Stress is a natural response of the body to various challenges in life. It is an inevitable aspect of life that affects everyone at some point. However, when stress becomes chronic, it can have negative effects on the body, including an increased risk of developing cancer. Chronic stress has been linked to a range of physiological changes that can impair the body's ability to fight off diseases, including cancer.

In order to reduce the risk of developing cancer, it is important to manage stress effectively. *Here are some strategies for managing stress:*

Exercise regularly: Exercise is a great way to relieve stress and improve overall health.

Regular physical activity has been shown to reduce stress levels and increase the body's ability to fight off disease.

Practice mindfulness: Mindfulness involves paying attention to the present moment, focusing on your breath and your body, and accepting your thoughts and emotions without judgment. Mindfulness has been shown to reduce stress levels and improve overall health.

Connect with others: Connecting with family and friends can help you feel supported and reduce stress. Joining a support group can also provide a sense of community and help you manage stress.

Get enough sleep: Lack of sleep can contribute to stress levels and interfere with the body's ability to fight off disease. Aim to get 7-9 hours of quality sleep each night to reduce stress levels and improve overall health.

Eat a healthy diet: Eating a diet rich in fruits, vegetables, and lean protein can help reduce stress levels and improve overall health.

Seek professional help: If stress is affecting your quality of life, consider seeking help from a mental health professional. They can help you identify the root causes of your stress and develop a plan for managing it.

Incorporating these stress management strategies into your daily routine can help reduce the risk of developing cancer and improve overall health. It is important to remember that everyone responds differently to stress and what works for one person may not work for another. Experiment with different stress management strategies to find what works best for you.

E. Staying Active and Engaged

Staying active and engaged is an important part of the anti-cancer lifestyle. Regular physical activity and engagement in social and intellectual activities can have a profound impact on your physical and mental well-being, especially in the context of cancer.

Physical activity, such as exercise or simply going for a walk, can help to maintain a healthy body weight, boost your immune system, reduce stress, and even lower your risk of developing certain types of cancer. Furthermore, regular physical activity can also help you cope with the side effects of cancer treatment and improve your overall quality of life.

In addition to physical activity, staying engaged in social and intellectual activities is also important for overall well-being. Having a strong support system and participating in activities that you enjoy can help to maintain a positive outlook and reduce stress. This can be especially important for cancer patients, who may experience feelings of isolation and depression.

It is important to find activities that you enjoy and that are within your physical abilities. This can range from taking a yoga class to playing with grandchildren, from volunteering in your community to pursuing a new hobby. The key is to find activities that bring you joy and provide a sense of purpose.

In conclusion, staying active and engaged is a vital component of the anti-cancer lifestyle. By engaging in physical activity, building strong relationships, and participating in activities that bring you joy, you can improve your physical and mental well-being, boost your immune system, and ultimately enhance your chances of surviving and thriving with cancer.

Conclusion

The conclusion of "Anti-Cancer: The New Way of Life" is a powerful reminder of the importance of taking control of our health and adopting a proactive approach towards cancer prevention and treatment. The journey towards good health and wellbeing is a continuous one, and this book serves as a comprehensive guide for anyone looking to live an anti-cancer lifestyle.

One of the most important takeaways from this book is the power of a positive attitude. Research has shown that a positive outlook can help boost the immune system, reduce stress levels, and improve the overall quality of life. When it comes to cancer, a positive attitude can help patients cope with the physical, emotional, and mental demands of the disease, and enhance the effectiveness of traditional and alternative treatments.

The anti-cancer lifestyle is a holistic approach to cancer prevention and treatment, encompassing several key areas such as diet, exercise, stress management, sleep, and more. By embracing this lifestyle, we can optimize our health and reduce the risk of developing cancer. The book provides a comprehensive overview of the lifestyle, including practical tips and suggestions that can be easily incorporated into daily life.

Finally, this book serves as an encouragement for anyone on the journey towards good health. The journey can be challenging, but by adopting an anti-cancer lifestyle, and with the help of support systems and medical professionals, anyone can beat cancer and live a long and healthy life.

In conclusion, "Anti-Cancer: The New Way of Life" is a must-read for anyone looking to take control of their health and prevent or treat cancer. The book provides a comprehensive guide to the anti-cancer lifestyle, and serves as a source of inspiration and encouragement for anyone on the journey towards good health.

Appendix : Additional information

A. Resources for Cancer Patients and Caregivers
1. National Cancer Institute (NCI)
2. American Cancer Society (ACS)
3. Cancer.Net
4. CancerCare
5. National Comprehensive Cancer Network (NCCN)

B. Recommended Anti-Cancer Websites
"The Anti-Cancer Lifestyle" website (www.anticancerlifestyle.com)

C. Anti-Cancer Recipes
1. Green Smoothie Recipe
2. Quinoa Salad Recipe
3. Lentil Soup Recipe
4. Grilled Vegetable Skewers Recipe
5. Sweet Potato and Black Bean Enchiladas Recipe

D. Glossary of Cancer-Related Terms
i. Cancer
ii. Carcinogenesis

iii. Chemotherapy

iv. Radiation Therapy

v. Surgery

vi. Immune System

vii. Metastasis

viii. Chemoprevention

ix. Complementary and Alternative Therapies

x. Oncologist